DATE DUE

PENGUIN BOOKS

WHEN A WOMAN'S BODY
SAYS NO TO SEX

Linda Valins began her research on vaginismus in 1986 and has written numerous articles
on the topic. She has trained as a crisis counsellor with The Samaritans, and in 1990
founded Resolve, the first support group for
women with vaginismus. She lives with her
husband in London.

WHEN A WOMAN'S BODY SAYS NO TO SEX

Understanding and Overcoming Vaginismus

LINDA VALINS

PENGUIN BOOKS

PENGUIN BOOKS
Published by the Penguin Group
Viking Penguin, a division of Penguin Books USA Inc.,
375 Hudson Street, New York, New York 10014, U.S.A.
Penguin Books Ltd, 27 Wrights Lane, London W8 5TZ, England
Penguin Books Australia Ltd, Ringwood, Victoria, Australia
Penguin Books Canada Ltd, 10 Alcorn Avenue, Suite 300,
Toronto, Ontario, Canada M4V 3B2
Penguin Books (N.Z.) Ltd, 182–190 Wairau Road, Auckland 10, New Zealand

Penguin Books Ltd, Registered Offices:
Harmondsworth, Middlesex, England

First published in Great Britain as *Vaginismus: Understanding and Overcoming
the Blocks to Intercourse* by Ashgrove Press Limited 1988
First published in the United States of America in simultaneous hardcover and
paperback editions by Viking Penguin, a division of Penguin Books USA Inc. 1992

1 3 5 7 9 10 8 6 4 2

A NOTE TO THE READER
The ideas, procedures, and suggestions contained in this book are not intended
as a substitute for consulting with your physician.
All matters regarding your health require medical supervision.

Grateful acknowledgment is made for permission to reprint excerpts from the following
copyrighted works:
Understanding Women: A Feminist Psychoanalytic Approach by Luise Eichenbaum and Susie
Orbach. By permission of HarperCollins Publishers/Basic Books. *Shrinks, Etc.* by Thomas
Kiernan. By permission of Doubleday, a division of Bantam Doubleday Dell Publishing
Group, Inc. *A Dark Science* by Jeffrey Moussaieff Masson. Copyright © 1988 by Jeffrey
Moussaieff Masson. Reprinted by permission of Farrar, Straus and Giroux, Inc. *Hunger
Strike* by Susie Orbach. By permission of W. W. Norton & Company, Inc. *Medicine &
Culture* by Lynn Payer. By permission of Henry Holt and Company, Inc. *The Road Less
Traveled* by M. Scott Peck. By permission of Simon & Schuster, Inc. *The Bell Jar* by
Sylvia Plath. Copyright © 1972 by Harper & Row, Publishers, Inc. Reprinted by per-
mission of HarperCollins Publishers.

Library of Congress Cataloging-in-Publication Data

Valins, Linda.
When a woman's body says no to sex : understanding and overcoming
vaginismus/Linda Valins.
p.   cm.
"Penguin books."
Includes bibliographical references and index.
ISBN 0 14 01.4908 2
1. Vaginismus.   I. Title.
RC560.V34V35   1992
616.85'83—dc20   91–4278

Printed in the United States of America
Set in Bembo
Designed by Debbie Glasserman

*This book is lovingly dedicated to
my parents, Julia and Nat Bensusan,
and my therapist, Dr. M.S.L.*

*Our sexual lives are not normally
shared with our parents, and if not
for this book I might never have
shared mine. However, I felt that
part of the healing process for me
and for other women lies in writing
and in ending the silence around
vaginismus. I therefore acknowledge
and thank my mother and father, as I
know how difficult this may be for them.*

Then the stories of blood-stained bridal sheets
and capsules of red ink bestowed on already
deflowered brides floated back to me. I
wondered how much I would bleed, and lay
down, nursing the towel. It occurred to me
that the blood was my answer. I couldn't
possibly be a virgin any more. I smiled into
the dark. I felt part of a great tradition.

—From *The Bell Jar* by Sylvia Plath

FOREWORD

This is a fine book. And this is a brave book. With courage and dignity, Linda Valins invites us to explore an aspect of women's psychological and sexual experience that has remained hidden and misunderstood for centuries.

Vaginismus, the involuntary contraction of the vaginal muscles, affects an estimated 0.17 percent of women in the United Kingdom, 20 percent of the women reporting to the Masters & Johnson clinic in St. Louis and 40 percent of the women who are seen at the Center for Human Sexuality at the State University of New York Health Science Center in Brooklyn.

These are staggering statistics. Behind them, as Linda so movingly points out, are the stories of hundreds upon hundreds of women who suffer in many different ways. They suffer because they live in a society geared to heterosexual consummation. They suffer because their vaginismus may render them infertile. They suffer because medical practice has often ridiculed and abused them. They suffer because the so-called sexual revolution of the late 1960s has made it difficult to admit that one isn't "doing it," can't "do it." They suffer a double burden, first from vaginismus and then from the silence and shame that follows this misunderstood experience.

Linda Valins's hard-won, compassionate relationship with herself translates into her feelings of concern toward other women who have suffered or still suffer from vaginismus. In daring to write openly about vaginismus she provides a lifeline to those many women about a silent hurt that may have made them feel hopeless. But this is a book of hope. Sufferers, their partners, their friends, gynecologists, and psychotherapists have much to learn from the scrupulous research she shares here.

Rather than presuming that there is only one way to get through the problem, Linda Valins points out the various routes that might provide the right kind of help (including self-help) for individual women. But in educating the general reader about vaginismus she does more than that. She simultaneously educates the physician, the health practitioner, the psychologist, the psychotherapist, and the counsellor about the problem and about the kind of stance the woman with vaginismus may appreciate and find helpful. The knowledge she so sensitively presents in this book will undoubtedly mean that it will find its way into both the consulting rooms and the waiting rooms of gynecologists and psychotherapists throughout the United States and the United Kingdom. I hope that its presence will mean an opportunity for women to bring up with their clinician a subject that has remained taboo for far too long.

Vaginismus, Linda Valins concludes, is not so much about sexuality per se but about the meaning of intimacy, about conflicts concerning dependency, about issues of trust for the individual woman. Vaginismus is about the woman's relationship to her body, her self-esteem, her relationship to giving, to receiving, to desire, to entitlement, to wanting, and how these themes then become psychologically and physically expressed.

These themes have powerful personal, familial, and social origins. Overcoming vaginismus then is not simply about being able to experience intercourse without the fear of excruciating pain or anxiety, but about understanding ourselves as women, as daughters, as mothers who live in a culture where female gender still means that a woman's place is pro-scribed, limited, drawn. We live in a culture in which wom-en's needs and desires, their wishes to act in the world and in their personal lives in their own interests can conflict with internal restraints so powerful that guilt, confusion, and in-security may accompany them.

The prohibitions on women acting on their own behalves are so strong and so deeply internalized that breaking them feels dangerous, as though one is cast adrift, deserting a known self-image. And yet that is what a woman wishing to overcome vaginismus may have to do. She may have to discover a self beyond the image of femininity she has ac-cepted for herself, she may have to discover what her body's "no" is trying to say for her, what inner conversation the contracting muscles speak, and what saying yes to her own desire might mean.

Linda Valins raises all these issues as she situates vaginismus in its historical and cultural context. And she does this while honoring the unique experience of the individual woman. This is an important book for women who suffer with vag-inismus. It is an important book for all those who work with women in a medical or psychological capacity. It is an im-portant book for all of us, for it challenges our prejudices and makes us think anew about women and their sexuality.

—Susie Orbach
August 1, 1991

ACKNOWLEDGMENTS

I felt it important to write this book in a format which would allow both sufferer and specialist to address the reader directly; therefore, this book could never have been written without the input of many people.

First, for the person who never gave up, even when at times I wanted to: love, appreciation and thank you to my therapist.

Special thanks to Dr. Paul Brown, who read my very first manuscript and encouraged me to continue, and to Robin Campbell of Ashgrove Press in Bath, who had the courage and commitment to publish this book.

Thank you to Susie Orbach for helping me to understand the social influences on women's psychology, both through her writing and in person.

I am indebted to Dr. Leonard Friedman for his pioneering publication *Virgin Wives* (1962); and above all for his help, encouragement and suggestions regarding my final draft.

I am particularly grateful to the following for giving up many hours of their time, offering highly practical and relevant information based on many years of experience in the field: Dr. Paul Brown, Psychologist in private practice, London and Bath, England. Dr. Martin Cole, Director, Institute for Sex Education & Research, Birmingham, England. Dr. Katharine Draper, Institute of Psychosexual Medicine, London. Dr. Patricia Gillan, Psychologist in private practice,

London and Wales, England. Marianne Granö, Sexual Psychotherapist, The Swedish Association for Sex Education, Stockholm, Sweden. Dr. Anne Mathieson, Institute of Psychosexual Medicine, London. Dr. Kenneth Metson, Homeopath & Osteopath, Essex, England. Dr. Robin Skynner, The Group Analytic Practice, London, England. Dr. Robina Thexton, Institute of Psychosexual Medicine, London.

My appreciation and thanks to the following, who helped to produce this American edition: Suzanne Arms-Wimberley, Palo Alto, CA. M. Brownell Anderson, Association of American Medical Colleges, Washington DC. Dr. Jelto J. Drenth, Rutgers Foundation, Groningen, The Netherlands. Dr. Yehudi Gordon, M.D., Consultant Obstetrician & Gynecologist, The Garden Hospital, London, England. Dr. Jules Black, obstetrician & gynecologist, Sydney, Australia. Judy Norsigian, Boston Women's Health Collective, Boston, MA.

My sincere appreciation to the following for their help in many different ways, particularly with my research: Dr. Morag Bramley, Dr. Willeke Bezemer, Sexologist, Office for Birth Control & Sexual Problems, 's Gravenhage, The Netherlands. Dr. Richard Carvalho, Society of Analytical Psychology, London, England. Dr. May Duddle, Institute of Psychosexual Medicine, London. Dr. Judy Gilley, Institute of Psychosexual Medicine, London. Judith Green, Institute of Psychosexual Medicine, London. Dr. Keith Hawton, The Warneford Hospital, Oxford, England. Dr. Michael Heap, British Society of Experimental & Clinical Hypnosis, Sheffield, England. Dr. Helen King, Department of Classics, Newcastle, England. Dr. Rosemarie Lincoln, Institute of Psychosexual Medicine, London. Dr. Tom Main, Institute of Psychosexual Medicine, London. Prof. Dr. Herman Musaph, Psychiatrist & Psychoanalyst, Amsterdam, The Netherlands. National Association for the Childless, Birmingham, England. Michael Silverston, Commercial & Legal Information Officer, Camden, London, England. Dr. Robert

Smallwood, The Shakespeare Institute, Stratford upon Avon, England. Hester Solomon, British Association of Psychotherapists, London, England. Dr. Prudence Tunnadine, Scientific Director, Institute of Psychosexual Medicine, London, England.

I would like especially to thank and acknowledge Dr. Prudence Tunnadine, scientific director, Institute of Psychosexual Medicine, for guiding me to some useful medical contacts.

I offer special thanks to all those doctors and therapists listed in the Appendix who generously agreed to be included as contacts for women seeking treatment.

My deep gratitude goes to my family and friends, who gave me the space to share the fact of my vaginismus with them, and who offered invaluable love, support and phone calls, especially Andrea, Asher, Benig, Chana-Mina, Charles, David, Dawn, Deirdre, Elaine S., Elaine W., Hazel, Heather, Jane, Jim, Julia, Kieran, Leslie, Martin L., Mary, Meir, Michael, Nelson, Pauline, Raymond, Ruth, Sherry and Tony.

I am indebted to Martin Valins, who not only shared the pain with me, but also had to live with a workaholic writer. He read every single one of the drafts of the book and was my most constructive critic. I could not have written this without his constant love, which has seen me through.

Above all, my greatest debt is to the women who bravely came forward and shared with me what were often extremely painful experiences and memories. With the exception of Jan, they have requested they be given pseudonyms for the purposes of anonymity. Thank you, Carol, Debbie, Emma, Frances, Helen, Jan, Jean, Naomi, Sarah and Valerie. This book is for you.

CONTENTS

INTRODUCTION

Somehow, even as a child, I always felt that I would not be able to have sex. This fear did not leave me and was brought into even sharper focus when I began to form relationships with men. It wasn't until my most committed relationship, which led to my marriage, that I summoned up enough courage to seek help.

Being able to have sex easily is taken for granted, and certainly for most of us the act of lovemaking is experienced as a natural, desirable and spontaneous part of life. But to women like me who suffer from vaginismus, this natural act is denied, resulting in nonconsummation of our sexual relationships and simultaneously depriving us of the opportunity to conceive children. I do not presuppose that penetration is a prerequisite for a loving sexual relationship, or that lovemaking can properly be defined as penetration. Many couples enjoy warm, loving sexual relationships without engaging in intercourse: these may include gay people as well as those who have physical disabilities. Furthermore, despite society's pressures, no woman should ever be made to feel that she is abnormal if she can't have intercourse, nor should she be forced into a sexual relationship. All of us should be free to find ways of affirming, celebrating and expressing our sexuality without needing to conform to rigid norms or fixed ideas about what sex should mean. We should all have a choice as to how we wish to make love. However, for the woman with vaginismus the choice of penetration is, because of the involuntary nature of the condition, not an option.

This book springs from the pain and loneliness I felt both before and during the time I was seeking help. Having vaginismus made me feel lonely, desperate, unsupported and isolated, as if I, and I alone, had this awful condition which nobody else knew about. They couldn't know about it, since it was rarely discussed on the radio and never on TV; it hardly appeared in agony columns; very little was written about it. So, I concluded, if nobody knew about vaginismus, who could possibly help me? In dealing with these feelings, I decided that one way of reaching other sufferers would be to share my experiences with them. In doing so, I hope that others may find the information, support and guidance which then seemed unavailable to me. I felt further inspired to write when I realized that if I had gone through such despair and misery, it was quite possible someone else had, too.

It has been difficult and often painful to write openly. So strong are internal and external pressures to make things appear "nice" and present my story with a smile that many times while writing I found myself wanting to protect the reader from the real pain and agony I went through. Although this book is intended to be positive, it must be said that the road to resolution is not always easy, and finding the right therapist may be equally difficult. Often the support and encouragement we may want or expect from friends, family and professionals is not available. It has been hard sharing my pain with people I know; it has been even harder sharing it in a book. However, the power and strength I have gained from these experiences lie within each and every woman who confronts her problem. Knowing this allows me to speak the truth without feeling compelled to protect and reassure the reader, or to suppress the realities about difficulties encountered.

I have been most strongly motivated by the work I have

been undertaking with my therapist over a period of more than six years, which has been the foundation of this book. Therapy has given me the courage to communicate how it feels to have vaginismus, as well as the knowledge that it can be successfully treated.

This book is partly my story; but I also discuss all the issues surrounding vaginismus as an essentially practical and empathic guide for any woman who thinks she may have vaginismus. I aim to remove the secrecy and shame surrounding vaginismus and thereby promote greater understanding among people in general, as well as among medical and sexual practitioners. I hope this will result in our being able to speak about any emotional problems freely and more openly. I address you as an individual, respecting your uniqueness. I hope you will use this book to help you make your own discoveries to lead *you* toward resolution. Above all, I want to be supportive, to encourage personal growth, and to assist in the realization of our potential, our power and our creativity, so that we can overcome our problems.

Vaginismus has been described as the Cinderella of women's sexual problems.[1] Concentration has been centered on birth control, abortion and choices in childbirth to such a degree that I feel a need to try and redress the balance. It would be comforting for us to walk into bookstores and see literature on vaginismus in addition to books on these other issues.

> I'm just so glad that someone is writing a book about this, as I feel that we are the forgotten few.
>
> —Valerie

I highlight the need for vaginismus to be recognized as an essential issue in women's health literature. Even more important is the need for a more positive and sensitive appraisal of the sufferer. During my research I was struck by the inaccuracy of some descriptions of both the condition and the sufferer. Many of the characterizations seemed stereotypical and damaging, reinforcing an already poor self-image. Words such as "frigid" and "childish" are not only negative but do not paint a true picture of a woman who has vaginismus. The majority of us are warm, loving and sensuous, consciously longing for intercourse but unconsciously fearing it.

Apart from Dr. Leonard Friedman's *Virgin Wives* (1962), there have been no books solely about vaginismus. While an excellent and concise study, *Virgin Wives* is thirty years old and is primarily a medical text. I was interested to see that the book closes with a plea that as vaginismus has never before been discussed at length it be further researched and more widely understood.

Is this book only for women who have vaginismus? No. While it's true that this book is about vaginismus, the causes and ways in which help can be sought are similar and equally applicable to any other emotional problem. This book will also have relevance to anyone who has either experienced or is experiencing difficulties in lovemaking or relating intimately, even though she may not have vaginismus.

This isn't a medical textbook, nor is it a sex manual; it is a personal statement. A simple but fundamental discovery I made is how important it is to love oneself and to feel loved in order to make love.

I hope that when reading this, you will be able to draw comfort from the knowledge that whatever fears, anguish or pain you may be experiencing, I have shared your feelings.

—Linda Valins
London, May 1988

WHEN A WOMAN'S BODY SAYS NO TO SEX

Chapter 1

LINDA

In describing my background I share with you a brief history of my family relationships. However, my background was not in itself a direct cause of my vaginismus. Instead, the way in which my particular psychology interpreted and coped with such events was the major factor in the condition's onset and development.

I was born on August 2, 1951, the eldest of four children, and was raised in a modest but comfortable rented terraced house in North London. My mother endured a long and difficult labor having me, and felt so disoriented that she was unable to notice the precise time of day I was born. She described me as a "beautiful baby who looked like a china doll." However, I did not sound like one, crying practically nonstop. My mother developed "milk fever" and was unable to continue to breast-feed, but I did not make the transition from breast to bottle with ease. My father often told me how he wore out a patch in the bedroom carpet from pacing the floor at night trying to get me to sleep. To this day I have problems falling asleep.

The house we lived in was shared by my mother's parents. Although unspoken, there must have been some tension in this arrangement. Conflicts must have increased when I was born, thanks to the unconscious competition over how best to raise me which was probably generated between my mother and grandmother. It must also have been difficult for my parents to freely express either anger or intimacy under the same roof as my grandparents. My parents tell me that as a little girl I was very loving, but extremely sensitive. At two years old, on a trip to the beach, I refused to put my bare feet in the sand and cried with fright until my shoes were put back on. From a very early age I was afraid of the water, and to this day I cannot swim.

My parents frequently told us they wished their lives had been different. Both had had opportunities to pursue careers in show business but for various reasons, including the war, had not been able to follow through. Consequently, they seemed to invest high hopes and expectations in all their children.

One of my earliest memories was at four years old, suddenly having to share my parents because of the arrival of a younger sister: my reaction is summed up by a family photograph taken two days after her birth, in which I am looking into the camera with tears in my eyes.

It was the mid-1950s, when preschool education was neither so available nor so widely accepted as it is today. I therefore spent the first five and a half years of my life solely in my family's company, with little outside contact. I was overprotected and, not surprisingly, on my first day at school the sudden separation from my mother was very traumatic. I felt shy and awkward with other children, and I recall my reluctance to go to their birthday parties. I would cry and plead with my mother to let me stay with her. The highlight of my elementary school days was the prospect of being met by my father after school. To me he seemed the tallest and handsomest of all the fathers, and my heart would leap when he peered through the glass panel of the classroom door to find me.

When I was six my brother was born. At the time of his birth I had measles and was therefore separated from him and my mother until I'd recovered. Looking back, I can see how this must have felt—to be separated from my mother when I was ill and needed her badly.

At home and at school I was always eager to communicate, and my teachers commonly criticized me for being too talkative. They referred to me on report cards as a "chatterbox." Although I enjoyed and excelled in art and English, my math was always very poor and I had a "can't do" attitude. I was terrified of anything competitive and consequently disliked —and was bad at—sports. This was in striking contrast with my mother, who had not only excelled in swimming as a schoolgirl, but had also been a team captain.

My feelings of exclusion began early, such as the times I stood at the edge of the pool watching my family swim, and on Guy Fawkes night when, afraid of the loud bangs from the fireworks, I remained alone indoors with my face pressed up against the glass, watching the rest of the family enjoy themselves.

When I had a problem, either personally or to do with school, I found it difficult to share it, since my parents tended to respond by getting overly upset. I then would feel compelled to comfort them, trying to reassure them that I didn't feel so bad. The most extreme form my trying to protect them took was when, at five, I developed an infection on my nailbed, possibly the result of intense nailbiting. Rather than tell anyone, I stood in an upstairs bedroom and cried silently with the pain. When I could endure it no longer, I finally showed my mother, but by that time it was necessary to have the nail removed at the hospital. I still recall the humiliation and shame I felt when the doctor and nurses admonished me for biting my nails. I felt as if I were to blame for the agony, as if I somehow deserved it.

A major trauma followed when I was nine years old, when my grandfather, whom I especially loved and who used to dress me for school, died of lung cancer. My grandmother and mother had nursed him throughout his illness, and I remember feeling repulsed by the blood and sputum in a bowl beside his bed. Although I wanted to mourn my grandfather's death, the air of stoicism in our household prevented me from crying openly. I had to suppress all my love and sadness.

In general, while anger was freely expressed among our family, there was little encouragement to show other feelings. I also had very little physical privacy, since I shared a bedroom with two siblings. Conversations in our house appeared to be uninhibited in their range of subjects, but in fact little was discussed at a personal level. Mealtimes were often noisy and chaotic, leading me to feel that my needs were not being individually acknowledged or met. My parents also accused me of being overly dramatic, but if that was true, it may have been the result of my feeling I was not being listened to; or perhaps I was merely emulating their overexcited responses. I often felt I was operating on a level different from theirs intellectually, that they were unable to participate in the kinds of discussions I wanted to have with them.

Nevertheless, my home was very much a warm, loving and "open" one, with people frequently popping in and friends often staying overnight. An important aspect of my upbringing was the tolerance, acceptance and generosity my family displayed.

I was very attached to my mother and admired her cleverness and her beauty. Although I wanted to be closer to her, I often felt she could not respond and in turn she did not acknowledge her own ability to love and to create. My father remained distant, an exciting but mysterious figure, simply because he was often absent, working seven days a week in a textile factory. This industry was known for its poor working conditions and intolerable deadlines. I sensed that he was tense and unhappy with his work but powerless to change his situation. The times we spent in each other's company my father was invariably exhausted, and he tells me how I sat quietly at his feet "allowing" him to nap in his chair.

Afterward he would praise me for not disturbing him. While I felt close and loving toward my sisters and brother, as the eldest I felt somewhat apart from them, often having to take on a bossy role which I resented and in which they still see me. Nonetheless, I have observed in comparison with siblings in other families how close and loyal we all feel toward one another.

My grandparents (particularly my grandmother) were my second parents. The boundaries between my parents' and grandparents' roles were blurred at times; it wasn't uncommon for me to eat supper with my parents and then go upstairs and have a second meal with my grandparents. Within this almost suffocating atmosphere I sensed how entwined we all were with one another. This extended to my mother's reliance on her mother; she seemed constantly to seek her help and approval. While in some ways this relationship was supportive, I came to realize that in other ways it was not very healthy.

I sensed that my parents felt torn between wanting to break out of the conformity of their generation and express themselves fully, and paradoxically needing to appear like everyone else in their close-knit community. In many ways my parents were quite unconventional, even wacky. I remember when I was twelve coming home from a friend's house to find my parents dancing the "Twist" with the record player turned up to full volume. This was a side of them which rarely showed itself.

The issues which seemed outwardly important to my family, but which conflicted both with my ability to be my true self and with my parents' to be theirs, included: conforming socially, appearing happy to outsiders, attending family functions even when we didn't want to, doing and saying the right things even when we didn't feel them, avoiding looking at inner conflicts, and pleasing others, even if it meant upsetting ourselves. If I had to summarize how I felt as a small child, it might read something like this:

I can't do it . . . No one understands me . . . I feel scared
. . . I feel so excited . . . I love Mom and Dad . . . I'm so
shy . . . It's all my fault . . . I hate everyone . . . I feel ashamed
. . . I feel alone . . . Am I loved?

When I was fourteen my mother gave birth to my youngest
sister. I felt a mixture of emotions: shame and secret envy of
her pregnancy as well as elation at the thought of a new baby.
I tried to conceal my mother's condition from school friends,
but when they found out many made fun of me. At the same
time my school also underwent dramatic changes, becoming
one of the first in the United Kingdom to go comprehensive
(encompassing ages eleven to sixteen). All my teachers left,
and I felt abandoned and alienated among children who
seemed little like me. Many of them seemed to be juvenile
delinquents, and some, as young as fourteen, were pregnant.
There seemed to be nobody I could trust, and I would often
be punched and bullied because of the "posh" way I spoke.
During this time my escape from misery was to mother my
newborn sister. I would often gladly step into my mother's
role and try to take care of the baby and of my father. To
protect my parents from the difficulties I was experiencing,
I felt compelled to keep my problems to myself.

My periods began late, at fifteen, and before they started
my mother was so anxious she took me to our doctor to see
if anything was wrong. Nothing was, but the idea of inserting
tampons terrified me. When my periods finally began I told
my mother. She responded with the Eastern European Jewish
custom, briskly slapping me on my cheeks to bring color to
my face. She then congratulated me. I was totally confused
by the slap and the congratulations. My mother had greeted
my womanhood with an apparent act of violence which made
me feel as if I'd done something wrong. This is not to say
there is anything deliberately sinister in this custom, but remember how sensitive a girl I was.

My periods made me feel embarrassed to be an adult and

ashamed that men might now find me attractive. I felt awkward when my parents complimented me on my growing body, and their remarks felt prurient and intrusive. My mother rarely spoke about sex and only briefly discussed how babies were made, but this conflicted with the sexual way in which my parents interacted with each other. They appeared to share private innuendos, and their sexual life seemed to me blatant because they'd created a baby in middle age.

Although considered bright by my head teacher and a candidate for university, I left school at sixteen with few qualifications. I finally trained as a secretary.

My training began in the world of TV advertising, where there was little sexual inhibition and illicit relationships among the staff were not uncommon. This was also the time of the Swinging Sixties, Beatlemania, the sexual revolution and the Pill. Here again, I felt apart . . . in conflict. Although I wanted boyfriends and had little difficulty getting dates, as soon as a boy sought an intimate relationship with me I became scared and withdrawn.

As I explained in the Introduction, I always felt I would not be able to have sex. But how, you may wonder, could a child know this? Perhaps this idea originally stemmed from the belief that I would never *become a woman* rather than never be able to have sex . . . the latter idea probably came later. Even at eighteen and nineteen, I still looked on as an outsider at other grown-ups, and this was finally encapsulated in my belief that I could never engage in the most adult of acts.

Throughout my late teens I had a series of boyfriends, but my fear of lovemaking was now so strong that the relationships inevitably ended. In common with many people of my generation I spent a large part of my twenties traveling to different parts of the world, but I never escaped the mystery deep inside me. No matter how many people I met or became close to, I never felt able to reveal this pain. When I returned to London I resumed secretarial work; although I received praise from employers, I never felt fulfilled in this role. Most of my friends were in professions, but I had the same "can't do" attitude when they asked why I didn't pursue a professional career. I was twenty-two when I met my husband-to-be, and he was the first person I could tell that I was frightened of intercourse. He listened and didn't laugh or reject me. It was his later support and encouragement which finally led me to seek help.

Today I feel as if I am more open as a person and, more important, I am beginning to know and understand myself. I hope you, the reader, will get a sense of who I am and how I feel from this and the forthcoming chapters.

Chapter 2

WHAT IS
VAGINISMUS?

It was by reading books like Dr. David Delvin's *The Book of Love*★ and *Treat Yourself to Sex*★ by Paul Brown and Carolyn Faulder that I discovered the problem I was suffering from actually had a name: vaginismus. Up until that time no doctor had made this diagnosis. This demonstrates not only how difficult it was for me to seek help, but also how difficult it was for doctors to help me. Jean had almost thirty years of suffering before she was told she had vaginismus:

> Since the 1950s I've had no end of treatments, but . . . only last year when I saw a new therapist did anyone tell me what was wrong with me.

> —Jean

THE CLINICAL DEFINITION

Vaginismus is an involuntary spasm of the muscles surrounding the vaginal entrance which occurs whenever an attempt is made to introduce any object, including a penis, into the vagina. Generally the spasm is limited to the vaginal opening, but many women also suffer from spasms of the muscles of

★ See Suggested Reading, page 349.

the thighs, anus, abdomen and buttocks. Each muscle or group of muscles can come into a state of spasm during attempted or anticipated intercourse.[1] Vaginismus isn't a disease, nor is it a physical disability. It is an emotional condition, the causes of which are psychological but which manifests itself in a physical response. Consciously we very much want to experience penetration, but deep down we are saying "No!" The unconscious muscle control of the vagina takes over from the conscious mind whenever intercourse is attempted.

Doctors refer to two types of vaginismus. The first (primary) vaginismus exists when a woman has never been able to tolerate penetration and the vaginismus has been present in every sexual relationship. The other type (secondary vaginismus) occurs in a woman who has previously enjoyed intercourse and then develops the condition after, say, a trauma. Doctors also differentiate between nonselective vaginismus (when the spasm appears with every partner) and selective vaginismus (when it appears with a specific partner). Furthermore, vaginismus is sometimes distinguished from apareunia, which means that the woman is able to insert her fingers or a tampon into her vagina but is unable to have intercourse. For the purposes of this book, however, vaginismus and apareunia will mean the same.

There are varying degrees of vaginismus, ranging from an occasional mild spasm to a very severe one:

> Even now you get some of the young senior house officers [residents] in gynecology who find it annoying when they're doing postnatals, and here's this woman, she's had two babies and she's still difficult to examine. You get a lot of middle-grade vaginismus, not total vaginismus, which causes pain and women get tense, it puts them off sex but it isn't that absolute total barrier that it can be for some women.
> —Dr. Katharine Draper,
>   member, Institute of Psychosexual Medicine, London

Although vaginismus is commonly referred to as a sexual problem, this isn't necessarily the way all therapists define the condition:

> Whether vaginismus is to do with sexuality is not for me a closed issue. There's an assumption that it's about sexuality, but I would be inclined to take a different starting point. It might be more about a woman's emotional receptivity having been damaged in some way because of what's been learned in the very early family history.
> —Susie Orbach, psychotherapist, London

Defining vaginismus is by no means a black-and-white issue. Indeed, the term can be used more loosely by doctors than the way in which I have defined it. In this way vaginismus is seen purely as a description of a symptom; neither a condition nor a diagnosis, but rather a way of describing what happens when a doctor tries to examine a woman's vagina. To use the word "vaginismus" simply to get a woman referred for treatment may not always be appropriate, because in some instances a woman's reluctance about being examined may be perfectly normal and she may merely need some reassurance to overcome the difficulty.

OUR PERSONAL DEFINITIONS

> Vaginismus is a medical term for a lot of pain, a lot of suffering and a lot of humiliation.
> —Jan

Medical definitions are not personal definitions. They are purely clinical and do not describe or convey vaginismus in terms of what it means for each of us. For me, vaginismus is a total blocking of all possibilities. That is to say, at its most destructive and powerful the spasm would occur vaginally, preventing me from being penetrated and creating new life. But vaginismus was not confined to my vagina. It also came into operation on other levels. It blocked my relationships with people by preventing me from opening up and trusting; it blocked my creativity, making my artistic abilities and imagination unavailable; it blocked me intellectually, rendering my power of mind unavailable and preventing me from pursuing a career.

Vaginismus is a term we can apply to many processes within us. For Sarah, it meant absolute fear. She likened it to being held back at school: "It held me back in every aspect of my life." It was as if she continually failed in one vital subject, and no matter how good she was in all the others, being hopeless in this one crucial subject prevented her from getting into any job or other endeavor in life.

Another sufferer, Jan, defines her vaginismus as "a closing off and shutting down of myself against the outside world."

Although vaginismus manifests universally as a vaginal spasm, it nevertheless can result from a diversity of conflicts, the origins of which may range from psychological to social. Each woman's vaginismus, though resulting in the same symptom, will be as unique as its causes.

IS VAGINISMUS THE ONLY CONDITION WHICH PREVENTS PENETRATION?

No. There may be reasons for nonconsummation other than vaginismus, and often the explanation is simple.

FEAR AND INEXPERIENCE

While not actually having vaginismus, a woman may be tense and anxious about her first intercourse. Her partner might get to the vaginal entrance, whereupon she might flinch a bit, causing him not to push any farther for fear of hurting her.

Another simple reason for nonconsummation is that often neither partner realizes that one or the other needs to use a hand to guide the penis into the vagina.

PAINFUL INTERCOURSE

"Dyspareunia" is the medical term for painful intercourse. It is important not to confuse this condition with vaginismus because dyspareunia allows penetration, albeit painfully. It is usually caused by physical, not emotional, problems. If dyspareunia remains undiagnosed and untreated, the anticipation of pain during penetration induces muscle spasm as a protective reflex.

Even though most infections do not actually involve the vaginal entrance, the fact that an infection can make penetration painful may eventually lead to vaginismus. A psychotherapist suspecting infection can try to localize the pain through history-taking and then indicate to the person conducting the physical examination the areas to inspect most carefully.[2]

I haven't listed them all, but some causes of dyspareunia may be:

- congenital deformity of the vagina (including a rigid or impenetrable hymen)
- infections which lead to pelvic inflammatory disease, such as herpes, thrush or vaginitis[3]
- hormonal abnormalities caused by menopause or endometriosis
- trauma caused by brutal sex, or scarred stitching of the perineum (episiotomy) after childbirth or female genital mutilation (clitoridectomy)
- allergic reactions or hypersensitivity to contraceptives or the lover's sperm

- tumors of the cervix, uterus, bladder or rectum
- insufficient lubrication as the result of inadequate foreplay or poor sexual technique

If the above are not diagnosed and treated, over the months or years intercourse can become increasingly painful and may result in vaginismus. Sometimes even after an infection has been cured a woman may still associate intercourse with pain. If medical examinations rule out any physical cause for the continuing pain, then, like vaginismus, dyspareunia may be considered psychological in origin.

Some women I talked with who do not have vaginismus tell me they dislike penetration because it feels invasive or painful. They confirm that there is nothing physically causing the pain but then go on to reveal how unhappy their relationships are with their partners. This leads me to conclude that painful intercourse may sometimes be a type of vaginismus in that the pain is being sustained psychologically, not physically. Dyspareunia can, therefore, be treated in the same way as vaginismus.

> Sometimes I've had a woman who has said she has difficulty with intercourse and I've examined her quite easily. But while she's been on the examination couch she has suddenly started talking about something that's bothering her, and you can feel the vaginismus develop on your finger. So it can be very variable according to what is actually happening.
>
> —Dr. Katharine Draper

IS VAGINISMUS A SEXUAL PROBLEM?

At first glance vaginismus may appear to be a sexual problem, since it clearly affects our ability to use our vaginas sexually. However, the origins of vaginismus do not lie in a woman's vagina or in her sexuality. They lie elsewhere, in the areas of:

- fear of intimacy
- fear of dependence
- lack of self-love
- poor self-esteem
- lack of trust
- feeling unentitled to needs

The reason that vaginismus is often felt and seen to be a sexual problem and thus mainly treated in a sexual way is simply because it *becomes* a sexual difficulty. However, the reasons that a symptom manifests in the vagina will be different for every sufferer. I therefore place vaginismus in a wider context so that the condition can be viewed outside our preconceptions about its relationship to intercourse, the vagina and the penis.

As psychotherapist Susie Orbach has explained, whether vaginismus has to do with a woman's sexuality is not a closed issue. It may have far more to do with a woman's emotional, not genital, receptivity. Sometimes dealing with vaginismus exclusively at a sexual or genital level can be somewhat of a red herring, leading both sufferer and therapist into a less effective understanding and less complete resolution. It may, for example, unnecessarily involve examining the partner's sexual potency as well as offering sexual techniques and vaginal gadgets aimed solely at achieving penetration.

As Dr. Willeke Bezemer, a Dutch sexologist, explains in her 1987 paper on vaginismus, an enlightened therapist would argue that treatment which results in a woman's explicitly not wishing penetration is as legitimate as treatment which ends in a woman's desire for intercourse being satisfied.[4]

When sufferers reveal their ideas of what penetration represents and why they feel unable to allow it, their comments indicate the depth of what intercourse means. Frances explains how vaginismus relates not to sex itself but to fears about intimacy and her inability to feel loved:

In sex I give myself and take in the man. To give and accept everything that oneself and the other person is seems to me a huge, monumental act that's also very ordinary. I always feel when attempting to make love that my deepest self is inside me and I'm not at all sure that who I am is known, loved and accepted.

WHEN WAS VAGINISMUS FIRST IDENTIFIED?

An important and comforting discovery for me was that I didn't personally invent vaginismus: it is a condition one develops. Therefore, there must always, throughout the ages, have been women who suffered from it. After understanding the ways in which *I* developed vaginismus I saw that the causes are not unique either to me or to any other woman in past or contemporary society. Indeed, vaginismus can develop in any woman regardless of age, color, class or culture. Vaginismus existed in women before you and me. We are not the first, and we are definitely not alone.

The earliest medical reference can be traced to Quincy's *Lexicon Medicum*, published in London in 1802. Suggested treatments around this time were always surgical, because psychotherapy did not exist. Thankfully, entries in recent medical dictionaries concentrate on the possible psychological nature of vaginismus and no longer suggest surgical treatments. Other references dating to 1880 are also found in homeopathic medical textbooks. It is a paradox that the more conventional medical literature affords comparatively little information about vaginismus, whereas unorthodox medicine devotes numerous pages to listing myriad remedies.

The term "vaginismus" apparently originated with a Dr. Sims, an American gynecologist during the 1860s.[5] He was the first to describe the condition, at a meeting of the Obstetrical Society in London in 1861. Further reference is made to vaginismus by Havelock Ellis (1859–1939), a British physician specifically interested in researching sex, relating to a case study in 1896.[6]

The greatest contributor to the study of twentieth-century sexuality was undoubtedly Sigmund Freud (1856–1939). As a psychiatrist practicing in Vienna, Freud introduced the concept of association between mind (psyche) and body (soma): hence "psychosomatic." As a treatment, psychoanalysis has direct relevance to vaginismus, since the condition is psychosomatic, induced by deep-rooted fear and anxiety. Vaginismus clearly demonstrates a woman's unconscious use of her body to express that anxiety, and a psychoanalyst would aim to discover the link between the present symptom and past experiences. Freud used techniques designed to reach the unconscious, as he believed problems can most effectively be resolved through the exploration and mobilization of repressed infantile experiences.

Reflecting the patriarchal era he lived in, Freud's work focused primarily on male psychology and sexual behavior. He seemed to profess ignorance about vaginismus, but did discuss the condition with his former pupil and colleague Karl Abraham during correspondence in 1924.[7] Despite the hostility and disgust that some of Freud's theories aroused (notably his discovery of infantile sexuality), the concepts and techniques he developed still influence the majority of today's therapies, many of which are used to treat vaginismus.

It was not until the study of sexuality was popularized in the late 1950s by Dr. William H. Masters and Dr. Virginia E. Johnson, the renowned American sex researchers, that vaginismus gained more prominence as an identifiable and treatable condition. Masters and Johnson are seen as the pioneers of sexual therapy, which, following their radical studies of female sexual response, became a major treatment for vaginismus (more about this and other methods in Chapter Five).

VAGINISMUS IN THE MOVIES

Although the term "vaginismus" has to my knowledge never been explicitly used in a movie, the condition has been alluded to.

Alfred Hitchcock's 1964 thriller *Marnie*, starring Tippi Hedren, tells the story of a woman unable to have sexual intercourse as a result of having witnessed and taken part in the self-defensive killing of her mother's lover. Marnie's childhood trauma has intensified her relationship with, and longing for, a mother who cannot love her properly. Interestingly, the film has Marnie's employer-turned-husband (played by Sean Connery) attempting to cure her of her sexual "block" with a quasi-psychoanalytic approach: he takes her back to her childhood to relive her trauma.

Ingmar Bergman's 1976 film *Face to Face* tells the story of Dr. Jenny Isaksson (Liv Ullmann), a psychiatrist suffering an emotional breakdown. Although not vaginismic, Jenny experiences intense muscular spasms of her vagina during an attempted rape, and about twenty-five minutes into the movie is seen describing this to a friend.

VAGINISMUS IN LITERATURE

It is interesting to note that Shakespeare's Ophelia is blamed by Hamlet for not consummating their love affair. She apparently has some sort of sexual conflict which could very well be vaginismus.

The novelist Sylvia Plath gives an account in *The Bell Jar* of the heroine, Esther, hemorrhaging during her first traumatic experience of penetration.

How often does the heroine in romantic novels and films whisper to her lover as she is about to be "taken": "Darling, be gentle with me"?

I keep wanting to change the ends of novels by putting the women into therapy.

—Dr. Katharine Draper

Somewhere there is an unspoken, unconscious fear of pain around allowing someone inside us, common to all women, and enough so for it to be alluded to in literature.

In their paper "Dyspareunia and Vaginismus" Dr. Philip Sarrel, Lorna Sarrel, and Dr. Carol Nadelson assume that all females feel a degree of penetration anxiety from childhood on. Without this assumption, they find it very difficult to explain women's extreme sensitivity to life experiences associating pain or difficulty and vaginal penetration.[8]

And we mustn't forget all the childless royal couples in fairy tales who are magically presented with a longed-for baby. Doesn't this eerily echo some of the psychological conflicts of women who cannot tolerate penetration and are desperate for a child? Perhaps the appeal of myths and legends lies in the way unconscious fantasies related to a developing child are represented in these stories.[9]

Outside the traditional medical literature, vaginismus has come to my notice in just three books to date. The first, an English book called *A Crying Game* by Janine Turner, tells the true story of a battered wife who suffers from vaginismus. The condition is specifically mentioned and its symptoms and causes described in the course of the painful account of a violent marriage.

The second is, surprisingly, a Japanese detective novel— *The Lady Killer* by Masako Togawa. It tells the story of Mrs. Taneko Honda, a woman whose husband has taken lovers because she suffers from vaginismus. Taneko's revenge— since she is unable to take lovers herself—is to kill her husband's mistresses and frame him for their murders. It is a frightening tale in which the desperation of a vaginismus sufferer is dramatically symbolized by a woman driven to murder.

The third, and most disturbing, book is *A Dark Science* by Jeffrey Moussaieff Masson, which includes a shocking account of a vaginismic woman's abuse by her physician.[10] It reads like a Gothic horror tale. Titled "The Amputation of the Clitoris and the Labia Minora: A Contribution to the Treatment of Vaginismus," the account explores the long tradition of male doctors operating on organs exclusive to women in order to cure their "hysteria." Other doctors acted by confining women whose imaginations they did not approve of to insane asylums.

We are told about J.P., a twenty-five-year-old single woman diagnosed by Dr. Gustav August Braun (a Viennese doctor born in 1829) as having vaginismus. His initial method of treatment is "to cauterize a good part of the labia minora." The foreskin of J.P.'s clitoris was also cauterized. This "surgery" was performed on November 11, 1864. On November 12th "a somewhat smaller lever pessary was inserted into the vagina, and vaginal pain did not occur. On 20th November the pessary was reinserted and then removed after two days because of increased irritation." Some time later J.P. was subjected to the amputation of her clitoris.

Masson concludes that whatever struck Braun as unusual, unattractive or threatening (he considered J.P. to have an overactive sex drive) was taken as a sign of degeneracy and therefore must be cured. Her supposed sexual arousal during the operation (Masson also suggests that Braun masturbated J.P.) only confirmed for the doctor the necessity of the surgery. Masson points out that fantasy played a considerable role in the minds of Braun and the physicians involved in J.P.'s treatment. He implies, as a warning to increase the consciousness of male physicians and female patients today, that these nineteenth-century doctors were somehow encouraged by the patriarchal society they lived in to carry their fantasies into direct action. (For further discussion of female genital mutilation, see Chapter Three, page 79; vaginismus and hysteria page 90; surgical treatments, see Chapter Five, page 178.)

IS VAGINISMUS RARE?

No. I would say that in any group of ten doctors there won't be many who won't have encountered vaginismus.
—Dr. Katharine Draper

One consumer guide on therapies reports that every sex therapist has seen at least one couple whose relationship has not been consummated because of vaginismus.[11] This must be quite a few couples!

Although much of the discussion about vaginismus centers around the extreme case in which a wife remains a virgin, this may represent only a small proportion of women who experience pain with penetration. As one psychiatrist points out:

If one includes mild as well as moderate and severe cases, then the prevalence must be much higher than if one restricts the definition to the situations in which vaginal penetration is impossible.
—Dr. Harold I. Lief, M.D., professor emeritus of psychiatry, University of Pennsylvania, and psychiatrist emeritus, Pennsylvania Hospital

One American study states that many more women report having had similar (vaginismic) experiences during periods of stress and marital difficulty. When viewed in this broader context, vaginismus is a much more common occurrence.[12]

I tend to see more vaginismus because I do referral clinics. During one year I do approximately two hundred and sixty-four, that is, approximately five psychosexual clinics per week. I think perhaps fifty percent of all patients have vagi-

nismus. I also do family planning clinics and meet vaginismus
often enough. . . . there might be one in a session of twenty
women.

—Dr. Robina Thexton, member,
Institute of Psychosexual Medicine

A disproportionately small amount of material is published
on vaginismus in relation to other female sexual problems.
Some books devoted to female sexuality don't even mention
the condition! Why is this?

Perhaps it's easier to write about men's problems as they are
discussed in technical terms. Women's problems, like vaginismus, are put in terms of feelings and not just technical
happenings.

—Marianne Granö, sexual psychotherapist,
Stockholm, Sweden

One reason for the continuing lack of accessible information since the publication of *Virgin Wives* might lie in the
misconception that vaginismus is a rare condition. While
not yet part of our everyday language, vaginismus has
nonetheless generated a whole series of medical papers in
countries as diverse as the Soviet Union, Bulgaria,
Poland, Czechoslovakia, Ireland, Sweden, Denmark,
France, Germany, Holland and Australia, as well as in the
United Kingdom and the United States.[13] In addition, a
Dutch sexologist gave several lectures on vaginismus at the
eighth World Congress of Sexology held in Heidelberg, Germany, in June 1987. Vaginismus is, therefore, a global
concern.

Confusion about its rarity seems to arise from a con-
tradiction: some medical texts suggest it is uncommon,
while others say it isn't and that the apparently low incidence is not so much evidence of the low number of sufferers as of the small proportion of women who come
forward.

Because we can't come forward and say we have vaginismus it's not thought to be a priority and gets pushed into the background.

—Sarah

This underlines the dangers of taking statistics at face value.

U.S. STATISTICS

Statistics, however impressive, can never convey the years of concealed anguish or the intensity of pain and despair that vaginismus causes every one of us. We need to remember this when considering the following:

- Approximately 20 percent of the women seeking help at the Masters & Johnson Institute in St. Louis have a demonstrable degree of vaginismus. (These patients originate from all fifty United States and from more than thirty other countries.)★

- "In my own research with my own clinic patients it runs around two percent," says Dr. Harold I. Lief of the University of Pennsylvania. "However, if I were a gynecologist doing sex therapy I have no doubt it would be much higher, say four percent."

- "Approximately forty percent of the women that we see here have vaginismus," says Dr. Marian E. Dunn, Ph.D., director of the Center for Human Sexuality, State University of New York Health Science Center, Brooklyn.

- Dr. Domeena Renshaw, M.D., director of the Sexual Dysfunction Clinic at Loyola University in Chicago, states that their vaginismus incidence rate is 7 percent, of which about one-third have a remedial physical basis.

★ Confirmed in a letter to the author from Dr. William H. Masters, Director of the Masters & Johnson Institute, dated October 1, 1990.

Statistics Outside the United States

Because of the nature of vaginismus, it will always be difficult to assess actual numbers. Therefore, I include British and Irish statistics because they further support the likely incidence of vaginismus throughout the United States and the rest of the world:

- Approximately 0.17 percent of women between fifteen and sixty-four (more than 27,200) in the United Kingdom alone are estimated to suffer from vaginismus.[14]

- There is a higher incidence (0.49 percent) among women between fifteen and twenty-four, representing the usual period of a woman's life when she first attempts intercourse.[15]

- One study reveals that women of all ages are statistically more at risk of developing vaginismus than they are of having to seek an abortion.[16]

- One doctor specializing in sexual problems estimates that vaginismus occurs in approximately 5 out of every 1,000 marriages in Ireland.[17]

- Another survey reveals that 16 out of every 100 women consulting one birth control clinic were suffering from vaginismus.[18]

- Between April 1986 and April 1987, in response to requests from readers, a leading newspaper's agony column sent out 1,000 leaflets on vaginismus, compared with 1,500 leaflets on how to enhance lovemaking.[19]

- Out of the total number of diagnoses made over a three-year period in the sex therapy clinics of Relate Marriage Guidance (a national bureau which offers marriage therapy), approximately 7 percent of the diagnoses were vaginismus. In the same period about 300 cases of preorgasmic problems were seen, compared to about 150 to 200 cases of vaginismus.

Why, then, is vaginismus apparently locked into a cycle of misconception about its rarity? Part of the reason might be an unwillingness on the part of the sufferer to come forward. Shame and loneliness combined with lack of information and confusion over how to seek help contribute to the condition's remaining unreported and untreated.

Vaginismus goes undiagnosed by doctors because of inadequate training. One study reveals that a woman had had extensive investigations for infertility before the fact of nonconsummation was elicited.[20] Two doctors, an ocean apart, point out how vaginismus often gets overlooked in their countries. In Britain:

> An increasingly common method of a woman coming for help was that she had been through everything to do with fertility investigations, often for several years, and then somebody had asked her whether she was having intercourse. It's often found out very late on in fertility clinics that the couple are not in fact having intercourse.
>
> —Dr. Paul Brown, consulting clinical psychologist

And in the United States:

> We have no concept of the national incidence of vaginismus. However, it is important to emphasise the fact that vaginismus is in all probability the most overlooked diagnosis, especially in gynecology. This statement particularly applies to the more moderate degrees of distress in given patients.
>
> —Dr. William H. Masters, M.D., director, Masters & Johnson Institute

Women who seek help for vaginismus often seek it from various sources and in a variety of places, namely via the general practitioner, family planning clinic, gynecologist, psychologist, psychiatrist, sex therapist, psychotherapist, psychoanalyst, hypnotherapist or marriage counselor. With no centralized coordinating body collating statistics on vaginismus nationally, this means the statistics available are often fragmented, difficult to interpret or out of date. Because they are largely incomplete, they do not give vaginismus the recognition and prominence it deserves.

A further impediment to collating statistics is the fact that vaginismus is a variable and not always permanent condition, occurring as it sometimes does after a specific event or untreated infection. Since it can develop in any stage of a woman's life, the number of sufferers is constantly in flux and, therefore, difficult to assess accurately.

These factors, combined with other issues discussed later in this chapter, all result in the myth that vaginismus is not only rare, but too rare to warrant serious attention.

> I think doctors have got to take vaginismus pretty seriously. People who say that it isn't a very big problem are just shutting their eyes to it.
>
> —Dr. Robina Thexton

HOW DO YOU KNOW IF YOU HAVE VAGINISMUS?

I am like all women who have vaginismus: anatomically normal, no different from any other woman. While unable to have intercourse, women who have this condition are nonetheless sexually responsive and very much long to make love. Though we fear penetration, we are still capable of sexual arousal and orgasm. Indeed, vaginismic women and their lovers often report a rich and varied sex life.[21]

> There's a myth amongst the general public that there's no sex when a woman has vaginismus. In fact, very many women who have vaginismus are really quite sexual. Not only are

they orgasmic when their partner stimulates them, but they
also are orgasmic during self-stimulation.

—Alison Clegg, sex therapy training officer,
Relate Marriage Guidance, Rugby, England

EXPERT CONFIRMATION OF SELF–DIAGNOSIS

The following is not meant to teach you how to diagnose
your own vaginismus, but rather to help you take the first
step toward arranging an initial consultation with a doctor
or therapist. Regardless of any suspicion either you or a therapist may have, an accurate diagnosis of vaginismus cannot
be established without the specific evidence gained from a
pelvic examination. Even if an internal exam is not possible,
an intuitive doctor should still be able to diagnose vaginismus
from sensitive observation of the patient's behavior on the
examination table or inability to tolerate an internal exam.
Without this consultation, women risk being treated for vaginismus when the condition is not present or, conversely, the
correct diagnosis may be delayed because the existence of
vaginismus has not been suspected by a therapist.[22]

A firm diagnosis of vaginismus is not just for the woman's
benefit (she is often relieved that there is nothing physically
wrong with her vagina), but it is also important for the
therapist:

I don't like to start work with a woman unless a physical
condition has first been eliminated. A clinical diagnosis which
confirms there is no pathology therefore gives me absolute
confidence to encourage and enthuse the client that we both
can do it.

—Alison Clegg

PHYSICAL CLUES

Vaginismus manifests itself physically in a number of ways; perhaps you will recognize one or more of these symptoms. Of course, you may have others not included here:

- The muscles surrounding the vagina contract involuntarily and go into spasm if intercourse is anticipated or attempted.

- These same muscles contract, making it impossible to insert a tampon or allow an internal examination.

- If an attempt is made either to penetrate or examine the vagina, the muscles of the thighs, anus, abdomen and buttocks draw together. To escape the doctor's approach, a woman may arch her back and withdraw toward the head of the examination table.

Carol gives a graphic description of what happens physically when she tries to allow penetration:

> I was completely tense and he tried to enter me. The pain was incredible, that's the only word I can think of . . . it was like I was being ripped open and sandpaper was being used on me. Afterwards I cried uncontrollably.

PSYCHOLOGICAL CLUES

Other early indications, while not manifesting physically, can be described as fantasies, fears and feelings. These may emerge long before penetration is attempted and often remain deep inside us; we may find it difficult to express them clearly in words. Any one of the following *combined with involuntary spasm* might be an early indication of vaginismus.

Fantasies play a large part in the onset of vaginismus, and

you may recognize your own among the following, commonly expressed by sufferers:

- Fear and anxiety that the penis is too large for the vagina.

- Belief that the vagina lacks elasticity, is too small and tight, and therefore won't stretch to accommodate an erect penis.

A recent study on vaginismus found that women of small stature who viewed themselves as frail little girls often carry a distorted image of their bodies into adolescence and adulthood. They picture their vaginas as tiny and frail and see an erect penis, as well as a finger or tampon, as huge and threatening.[23]

This was confirmed when I met Sarah:

As a teenager I was so thin, I assumed my vagina must also be too small and tight.

- Association of penetration with pain and damage, imagining we'll be ripped or torn apart if entered. Because of this phobia, sexual contact which might lead to intercourse is often avoided.

- Acute anxiety about all the body's orifices, and a fear of touching our insides:

There are women who are frightened of any kind of penetration. One woman couldn't bear anybody looking at or touching her umbilicus. Others say they can't bear dental treatment either.

—Dr. Robina Thexton

- Strong negative feelings including revulsion toward the vagina and fear of looking at or touching it. This can compound our ignorance about where the vaginal opening actually is.

- Belief that we are cloacal: that is, possessing only one orifice through which we urinate, defecate and make love.

- Irrational fears about our bodies which bear no relation to fact and are not necessarily connected with inadequate sexual education: for example, fear that the penis will penetrate the abdominal wall and damage internal organs; imagining the vagina to be a bottomless pit that will swallow things up; confusing the vagina and rectum, imagining that a tampon or penis will go into the back passage by mistake:

One woman showed me that when she examined herself she could never find her vagina and I observed that her finger always slipped further behind. Then, during hypnosis, we were able to make the link that a man who had assaulted her when she was four had put his finger into her anus, and that had fixed her sexuality.

—Dr. Anne Mathieson, medical hypnotherapist

- Fantasies about the hymen which may be the result of partial intercourse, when the partner manages to penetrate a little but suddenly the vagina goes into spasm and prevents any further penetration. The woman then believes the penis is being blocked by an inner hymen which is high up inside. Other fears are that the hymen is still intact or so strong it has to be removed surgically before intercourse.

HISTORICAL CLUES

Many women have had a horrifying penetrative experience of another sort, such as a rectal biopsy or passing of a catheter into the bladder.

—Dr. Robina Thexton

My own findings are confirmed by Sarrel, Sarrel and Nadelson, who describe the childhood and adolescent events which may increase penetration anxiety. There are the nongenital experiences which involve repeated injections, unusually painful or frightening dentistry, frequent throat cultures or one or more urethral dilations done without anesthesia. In each case the little girl experienced a combination of pain and extreme anxiety. Other early experiences involved genital trauma, such as removal of a vaginal boil, accidental injury to the vulva (perhaps when riding a bicycle or climbing a fence), unusual pain and difficulty when inserting tampons (see page 72) and unpleasant pelvic examinations. It was found that in every case it is less the experience itself than the emotional climate surrounding it which matters. Variables in a girl's personality, her parents' ability to reassure or their tendency to overreact, attitudes of doctors, nurses or dentists involved, are all crucial.[24] So a woman may have any of a number of "historical" clues:

- female genital mutilation (ritual removal of the clitoris)
- initial painful or clumsy attempts at penetration
- sexual abuse or rape
- traumatic pelvic or rectal examination
- expectation of painful intercourse because enemas or soap suppositories were administered in childhood, causing pelvic pain

ARE WOMEN WHO HAVE VAGINISMUS ALL ALIKE?

There is no evidence that any one personality type or psychological disorder predisposes to vaginismus, although clinical evidence supports the suggestion that anxious and fearful women are overrepresented among vaginismus patients.[25]

> There is no true picture of a woman who has vaginismus
> . . . all are different.
> —Barbara Lamb, nurse-therapist,
> Parkside and Harrow College of Nursing & Midwifery,
> Harrow, Middlesex, England

Although we share the same symptom, we have to remember
that each of us is unique.

> With vaginismus, one is bracketing together events which
> have different causes, but are simply identified by the same
> symptom.
> —Dr. Martin Cole, sex therapist

The majority of doctors and therapists agree that it is very
important not to give sufferers more labels by saying they
are in a particular state for a particular reason. One therapist
pointed out that the meaning of a woman's vaginismus is
actually highly individual and private.

However, there is perhaps one common factor:

> The sufferers are very different from each other. Of course,
> I work all the time with the father-mother relationship in
> mind, but that's the only similarity.
> —Marianne Granö

THE CONSPIRACY OF SILENCE

How can a condition so serious and potentially widespread
remain comparatively unspoken and unwritten about? This,
too, in a society which seemingly promotes sexual freedom
in the media as often as our favorite recipes?

Or are we so sexually free? Sex still remains an emotionally
charged area for most of us, so it's easy to see why the very
nature of vaginismus makes it difficult to speak about. Talking about it means not only having to describe an intimate
act normally shared just with one's lover, but also having to
admit to its failure. Yet it is somehow more than that. It is

almost a conspiracy of silence because the difficulty in speaking about vaginismus is twofold . . . the silence is maintained not only by the sufferer but also by those around her.

HOW SEX IS PERCEIVED

Generally we are unable to speak honestly about sex, having to conceal inadequacy with bravado. So long as we attach shame to sexual problems or believe them and their sufferers to be rare, there will be no space in which little-known problems like vaginismus can be discussed. Denying that sex is commonly problematic inevitably leads to a failure to speak honestly about it.

Lack of respect for and honesty in talking about sex can make it impossible for families to communicate in a comfortable and natural way. This means that parents are often the last people to whom daughters feel they can talk about their vaginismus.

The essence of sexual expression is often lost in the deluge of information. With numerous books and radio call-in shows covering orgasm and obsessed with performance, positions, frequency and technique, sex is rarely spoken about except in these terms.

Heterosexual lovemaking is defined by penetration. This is demonstrated by the fact that a marriage can be legally ended if consummation has not taken place. Consequently, we feel vulnerable to exposure and ridicule if we reveal our vaginismus publicly.

THE MYTHOLOGY OF THE SEXUAL REVOLUTION

Psychotherapist Susie Orbach explains that she believes vaginismus might have been more common in the 1950s. When the so-called sexual liberation of the 1960s came into being, pretending to focus on sexuality but in fact focusing on *male* sexual liberation, it became inappropriate for women to admit to having sexual problems. In the late 1960s and early 1970s, when the focus moved to the clitoris, the emphasis shifted away from women who might have needed to talk about vaginismus, because the vagina was no longer central:

> Because the clitoris became the major sexual organ, conversation around penetration moved to the background. This meant that the focus moved to other issues of women's sexuality. With the focus removed from intercourse it then became somehow shameful for women who had vaginismus to even speak up and share their problem.
>
> —Susie Orbach

THE POTENTIAL POWER OF WOMEN

Anne Dickson, psychologist and author (*The Mirror Within*, 1982, and *A Woman in Your Own Right*, 1985; see "Suggested Reading," page 349) was trained in sexual counseling at the National Sex Forum in San Francisco. In 1980 she founded the Redwood Women's Training Association, which offers assertiveness training and courses in women's sexuality in the United Kingdom and Ireland. When we met during my research for this book she suggested very perceptively one of the reasons that vaginismus may be seen through the "collective male unconscious" as a symbol of power over men:

> Vaginismus is an uneasy reminder that women can say "No."
> A lot of men feel extremely uncomfortable about the power of the vagina. It's to do with their unease and discomfort about the potential ability of women to refuse. If we did exert this power in the outside world then the world might change, but we can't, so it remains an undercurrent.

I was reminded of Aristophanes' *Lysistrata*, in which the women choose to withhold conjugal privileges from their husbands until the men stop fighting in wars.

DOCTORS' UNEASE ABOUT VAGINISMUS

The silence may also be maintained by the unconscious reluctance some doctors feel to recognize the existence of vaginismus. Having to treat the condition may, for example, require a person to confront parts of himself or herself which are closed to love and openness. All of us, naturally, wish to avoid looking at these aspects of ourselves. Such unease may take the form of either unconsciously colluding with the woman to deny her problem (by sending her away with no treatment), or considering vaginismus purely physical. If doctors shout at us or send us away, perhaps they need to ask themselves what so terrifies them about vaginismus that they must do this. I believe it could be terror of their own closedness, or perhaps envy of the woman who is able to make some kind of protest.

NEGATIVE FEELINGS

Women who suffer from vaginismus may share a number of negative emotions that compound the conspiracy of silence.

- Further barriers to seeking help are fear of ridicule and loss of self-respect, created in part by the belief that revealing a sexual problem is admitting to failure.

- Owning up to being in a nonconsummated marriage carries with it the fear of being stigmatized by society as part of an improper or even unwholesome union.

- We feel compelled to conceal vaginismus lest we be seen as abnormal, partly because of our erroneous assumption that people who have sexual problems are somehow peculiar, in the minority, or can even be picked out in a crowd:

I was afraid everyone would laugh if they knew and I would never be able to face them again . . . it would be so humiliating.

—Sarah

People seem to be frightened of catching vaginismus . . . like a disease.

—Jan

The truth is that very few people go through life without ever experiencing a sexual difficulty. We only have to think of the man, the worse for drink or under stress, who can't get an erection . . . or the woman who experiences pain during intercourse after an infection, childbirth or marital conflict.

- Because cause and blame are so often mistakenly connected, we feel somehow to blame for failing in the deepest expression of physical love.

I still feel so guilty that for the first four years of my marriage I couldn't be more of a wife, as we never made love properly.

—Sarah

- The shame attached to vaginismus can make us feel alienated from all sexual activity, inadequate and fraudulent:

One woman told me for years she used to sit on the train and look at women around her and feel different and wonder why she couldn't be like the others.

—Barbara Lamb

I remember, before I went into therapy, desperately wanting to tell my problem to the first available stranger (at a bus stop or in a train station). Although it seems irrational now, at that time the only person to whom I could ever envision revealing my secret was a total stranger . . . someone anonymous whom I'd never have to see again. Because I so loathed my vaginismus I imagined everyone else would, too.

VAGINISMUS AND YOUR PARTNER

Vaginismus puts a great strain and distress on a relationship. A woman is battling with negative feelings about herself and a feeling of lack of success in life, which are always counter-productive to happiness.

—Dr. Robina Thexton

Having vaginismus affects all our relationships, but most of all it affects our relationships with our lovers. The effects can be far-reaching, since the severity of vaginismus results in nonconsummation of sexual relationships and marriages.

FEELING GUILTY

I'm eaten up with guilt about making my husband live a life without sex.

—Valerie

My husband and I are fortunate to enjoy a close, loving relationship and are able to share many things. Still, my inability to express my love for him in a physical way eventually led me to feel that I wanted to be free of him and the marriage. I saw this as a way of getting free from the pressure to resolve vaginismus. Since we could not have intercourse we couldn't make babies, and I would plead with him to meet someone else and divorce me, thereby releasing me from the guilt I felt at not being able to give him a child.

A BAN ON LOVEMAKING

We don't make love, but it's more than that because we don't come together sexually at all.

—Jan

Though it might seem too obvious to mention, the physical relationship between my husband and me also suffered. It's possible for a couple to maintain a good sexual relationship despite vaginismus, and for many years we did. However, as time passed and the vaginismus continued, our whole sexual life focused on penetration. At this point, sexuality and the hope of making love for the purpose of communicating were lost. I felt that unless I was penetrated any sexual contact was meaningless. Each time I set myself up for success . . . only to feel like a complete failure again.

As one sufferer points out, the mere expectation of the vaginismus is enough to set the reflex into motion:

If vaginismus happens once, you feel that it will definitely happen the next time, and the next. Consequently, it does.

—Carol

I finally concluded that *no* lovemaking had to be preferable to continual failures or sex without intercourse, and thereafter for long periods I imposed a state of misery on our marriage: celibacy.

It was almost like there was a deadly secret between us, and after a while we stopped trying to make love and never mentioned it.

—Sarah

My husband accepts the situation and we don't make any attempts at intercourse any more.

—Valerie

ENFORCED INFIDELITY

Waves of guilt and inadequacy washed over me because I was unable to have complete sex or to conceive a child. I would beg my husband to leave me for a woman who could manage to do both. In effect, I tried to push him into having affairs.

Although the vaginismus had been present in my previous relationships and I'd never been able to insert tampons, I began to fantasize that perhaps my vaginismus was continuing because I was with the wrong man. I then imagined taking a lover to test whether I would have the muscle spasm with him. Although I was able to work through this fantasy without acting on it, I can certainly understand why Jean felt compelled to:

> I tried having lovers, thinking it might just be the combination of my husband and me that stopped me . . . but it was the same. Both men said how very relaxed, responsive and sexy I was . . . but for all my responsiveness I still couldn't make love.
>
> —Jean

THE THREAT OF MARITAL BREAKDOWN

> Vaginismus caused the breakup of my first marriage, as it broke down all communication between my husband and me.
>
> —Sarah

When I felt my most wretched, hopeless and destructive, I wanted to end my life. I became unreachable and unconsolable, even by my husband. Needless to say, the consequence of this was a deterioration in our relationship, and we found ourselves in the midst of a marital crisis which compounded the severity of my vaginismus even further.

Masters & Johnson report that vaginismus can affect a man's sexual performance and that he may be unable to maintain an erection because of repeated failures at penetration.[26] Kaplan also reports that reflecting the cross section of relationships generally, the quality of vaginismic marriages varies considerably, ranging from excellent to deeply troubled.[27]

> However many couples we are talking about, there will be as many different effects.
>
> —Jill Curtis, psychotherapist

In the light of my own experiences and those of other sufferers, I would like to add that vaginismus places an extreme emotional and physical strain on *any* relationship, whatever the quality.

CAN YOU INHERIT VAGINISMUS?

> Women frequently say that their mother had this problem. She might say that her mother couldn't make love for quite a long time, "so I'm just the same as she was." She is almost accepting permission to have a problem so as not to be better than Mother.
>
> —Dr. Robina Thexton

I am the eldest of four, and neither of my two sisters has vaginismus. Vaginismus cannot be genetically passed down between parent and daughter simply because it is a condition a woman develops, not one she is born with. Nevertheless, it is possible for a mother with unresolved sexual anxieties to unconsciously transmit feelings to her daughter which can contribute to the onset and development of vaginismus.

> Women frequently say their mother doesn't enjoy sex. I've certainly had women say, "My sister had to have an operation before she could have sex."
> I was examining one girl who had vaginismus. She suddenly said to me on the couch, "My mother had a lot of problems with sex, but then she had a dream and she dreamt

that Saint-somebody-or-other was doing what you're doing now, and after that it was all right."

—Dr. Katharine Draper

In one case study it was reported that a vaginismic woman recalled that her own mother also had the condition and had difficulty tolerating full penetration to that day.[28] It would be safe to assume, therefore, that this daughter had psychologically inherited her mother's vaginismus in the same way a sensitive child might psychologically inherit her father's phobia of thunderstorms.

Though women haven't said their mothers or sisters have vaginismus, some mothers of vaginismic women seem to set up a model for psychological vaginismus in their daughters. One woman's mother would never confront any of the males in the family and would actually go out in the garden to get away from them if there was any trouble. In this case, the mother was setting up in a psychological way exactly what the sufferer is now doing in a physical way.

—Jill Curtis

My therapy revealed that this has more to do with a woman's emotional perception of her mother's anxieties and the way the mother transmits them than with any flaw in the mother's character, attitudes or personality. Any anxieties and attitudes communicated to us by our parents are totally unconscious, and this knowledge helped me to recognize that my parents did not knowingly cause my vaginismus.

CAN A WOMAN WITH VAGINISMUS CONCEIVE A CHILD?

Yes. In some instances vaginismus is only detected in the prenatal clinic or after delivery and is found not to improve after the birth of a child.[29]

VAGINISMUS AND INFERTILITY

I saw myself as infertile but considered myself dishonest for not revealing the true reason for my childlessness. I was hard on myself because, as I discovered in therapy, I felt undeserving of sympathy and comfort. That I felt I had to deny the truth of my "infertility" only added to my isolation.

> Medically, anyone who hasn't conceived in a certain amount of time is infertile, so we shouldn't isolate ourselves from what could be real support, even if the treatments are inappropriate. Every infertile woman's problem is painful to them, and everyone, to some extent, feels a "cheat" and a social stigma.
>
> —Emma

Unless a woman has gynecological problems, it can be assumed that the only relation vaginismus has to infertility is that it can prevent conception. Much of the anguish which surrounded my inability to conceive also stemmed from childhood feelings about an inability to be part of the adult world and bear my own children.

VAGINISMUS AND THE LAW

Legal history contains the 1926 peerage rights case of Christabel Lady Ampthill, wife of the third Baron Ampthill, who gave birth to a son, but not as the result of sexual intercourse.[30] Lady Ampthill admitted that she was a virgin and that no normal sexual intercourse had ever taken place during her marriage. Records confirm this: "[Christabel] admitted that her husband had never effected penetration and that he had been in use to lie between her legs with the male organ in more or less proximity to the orifice of the vagina and to proceed to emission . . ." There is even a legal term for this, "conception by *fecundatio ad extra*." Doctors call it "intracrural intercourse" when the partner ejaculates outside the vagina.

It is likely that Christabel suffered from vaginismus, and although that fact was never disclosed, the court recognized that a child can be conceived without penetration taking place and ruled in favor of Lady Ampthill, resulting in peerage rights being granted to her son.

IMPREGNATING ONESELF

> I think the request for AIH [Artificial Insemination with the Husband's sperm] is made quite often by women who desperately want a pregnancy and aren't able to have intercourse in the usual way.
>
> —Dr. Robina Thexton

The wish to become pregnant is understandable; for many women it is a natural longing. For the woman with vaginismus, the desire for a baby is sometimes so overwhelming that it can override the wish to accomplish intercourse. In his paper "Vaginismus and the Desire for a Child,"[31] Dr. Jelto Drenth points out that not all women experience nonconsummation as a sexual problem. Sometimes sex without intercourse is fully satisfying to the couple and their desire for a child is their only reason for seeking treatment. Consequently, consummation is neither the one and only treatment goal, nor sex therapy the only method.

> When I didn't think I was going to get over my vaginismus, and I wanted a child, I thought of asking for artificial insemination, but it never got any further.
>
> —Sarah

Another sufferer describes the longing to fill her internal void:

> I had to know that I was a real woman, that I wasn't frigid. I had to have a child so that I could be fulfilled, yet I couldn't have penetration.
>
> —Jan

The longing for a child is sometimes acted on with impregnation taking the form of one of three procedures:

- The partner ejaculates on the outside of the vagina (as in the Ampthill peerage case).

- The woman impregnates herself by injecting her partner's semen into her vagina with a syringe (not possible in the majority of women whose vaginismus is severe).

- A doctor injects the husband's semen into the woman.

Dr. Drenth states that AIH is an acceptable alternative for some women; if a couple is not interested in intercourse for sexual satisfaction but only to conceive a child, AIH may be considered. Sometimes, when therapy proves too much for the couple, AIH will become attractive to them at a later stage.[32]

DELAYED LABOR AND TRAUMATIC DELIVERY

Dr. Katharine Draper stressed to me that she believed it was particularly important for women who conceive despite their vaginismus to have treatment during pregnancy; otherwise the symptom will make the necessary examinations during delivery traumatic and may lead to a delayed labor.

> We had some women in our study who conceived through intracrural intercourse, and they hate the examinations. I think these women are the most urgent to be treated.

Hypnotherapist Dr. Anne Mathieson explains how she uses hypnosis to help the woman who has vaginismus through a subsequent labor:

I always say to a woman who comes to me with vaginismus that I'd like to see her when she becomes pregnant because pregnant women are particularly responsive to hypnosis. Suggestions can then be made concerning the confidence and relaxation needed for a good experience of pregnancy and childbirth and of successful breast-feeding if this is her wish. During pregnancy, suggestions can also be made that she will be able to relax and have the confidence to enjoy and express her sexuality fully when she feels ready for this after the birth of her child.

It has also been reported that vaginismus is frequently unaffected by the passage of the baby's head during delivery and that women with vaginismus who become pregnant find their spasms much more difficult to resolve once the much-desired pregnancy has been achieved.[33]

IS AIH THE ANSWER?

Opinions differ on the appropriateness of AIH for a woman who is not able to resolve her vaginismus. Dr. Drenth states that there is not much sympathetic support for women in the scientific literature when intercourse is not their treatment goal, and there seems to be almost no literature on this indication for AIH. He adds that it is strange, particularly in times of all sorts of high-tech assistance with fertility, that a pregnancy is almost never acknowledged as the true goal of therapy for some vaginismic women.[34]

Ultimately, the decision to have artificial insemination will belong to the couple and their therapist. Many therapists told me they would not stand in the way of a woman's choice to have a baby, despite the spasm:

If one felt this was a couple wanting a child and they'd approached treatment as honestly as they could, then I would support them in AIH.
                    —Dr. Paul Brown, consulting clinical psychologist

Nurse-therapist Barbara Lamb told me she felt particularly sensitive to a woman's desperation for a baby:

> I think it would be terribly cruel not to help her have a baby simply because she can't come to terms with her vaginismus.

However, sex therapist Dr. Martin Cole, while supporting AIH, is unsure about the long-term effects:

> I think AIH is a good idea, but I have some doubts as to whether a pregnancy helps the vaginismus.

The majority of practitioners told me that generally they would try to play for time and see if they could get intercourse going in the usual way, but that they would not rule out AIH.

Often one factor that prompts a woman to seek help is her longing for a child. In most sex therapy programs, the wish for a baby is discussed at the outset of treatment:

> One of the terms of our contract is that the clients should use adequate contraception during treatment. I spend quite a bit of time clarifying this, since clients with vaginismus often have come for help because they want a baby. It's extremely important they understand that starting a family before the sexual difficulty is properly resolved will almost certainly mean that the sexual relationship will continue to cause problems after the birth of the child.
> —Alison Clegg, sex therapy training officer,
> Relate Marriage Guidance, Rugby, England

BYPASSING A WOMAN'S SUBCONSCIOUS
TO ACT ON A FANTASY

Any concern I feel about AIH for a woman with vaginismus springs from my own experience and has not been influenced by doctors or books. Let me explain, then, why I believe artificial insemination would not have been appropriate for me, so that you can see the possible negative aspects of what may at first seem a shortcut to becoming a mother or to happiness. The practitioners who were opposed to AIH took this view simply because they were concerned for the woman's long-term welfare and not because of moral or ethical issues.

As two practitioners explain:

> The request for AIH isn't made very often, but on the whole I would personally be very reluctant because of the bypassing of psychological difficulties.
>
> —Dr. Katharine Draper

> I would be very worried about a request for AIH and my response would have to be "Hold still a moment." For me, it would mean that we've still got a lot of work to do.
>
> —Jill Curtis

Unconscious childhood fantasies which remain active in a woman's mind may be the real determinants of her wish for AIH.[35] If we take just one example: psychoanalysis of children confirms that a girl's discovery that she has no penis (penis envy) can feel so depriving that she may deal with it by denying the differences between men and women.

As I suggested earlier, a woman with vaginismus may use her own syringe to inseminate herself; in doing so she may be acting on an unconscious fantasy that there *is* no difference between men and women, and that she can therefore make herself pregnant without a man.[36]

During periods of utter despair, when I felt that my therapy would never help me and when my longings for a child overwhelmed me, I begged my analyst to arrange AIH or at least support me in the procedure.

At first, his refusal to help me arrange AIH seemed cruel, and I threatened to end my analysis. However, as I came to understand and work through these feelings I realized that his refusal to arrange artificial insemination was actually a loving act. We were able to explore the unconscious imaginings or fantasies behind my wish for AIH, and saw that it was based less on reality and more on the primitive fantasy that intercourse is not necessary to produce a baby. My wish for AIH represented a desire to magically be impregnated and to turn away from looking at the internal forces within which produced my vaginismus.

Again, psychoanalysis confirms that in order to deny the conflict-laden idea that parents have sex, children often imagine that something magical is done to Mother by a doctor to make her pregnant.[37] If my analyst had supported me in AIH he would have been colluding with me in acting out my unconscious fantasies. We both would have been taking my fantasy about not needing sex to produce a baby quite literally, and he would have unwittingly helped me bypass my real problems.

In looking at my own psychological development, I notice that women with vaginismus share an inability to separate psychologically from their mothers. If we don't experience ourselves as being separate from Mother, a request for AIH may be an unconscious attempt to get a baby from her.[38] This particular fantasy was very much alive inside me; many times I imagined that if I told my mother about my problem she could magically present me with a baby and "make it all better."

Echoing my own fantasies, Swedish sexual psychotherapist Marianne Granö is careful to notice a woman's inability to separate from her mother:

> If a woman's wish to tell Mother about the vaginismus is very strong, I always ask why. It may be the fantasy for Mother to help her with everything, so it's important to discuss it because we have to recognize how unrealistic it is when you're adult to talk with Mother about everything.

In trying to uncover the subconscious fantasies that might lie behind our wish for artificial insemination, I hope not to offend any woman who has conceived a baby through some other method than intercourse. My concern about AIH is for the woman who suffers from vaginismus, not for the woman who has physiological problems which prevent her from conceiving in the normal way. Most important, I do not wish to imply that women with unresolved vaginismus can never make good mothers, because of course they can. However, muscle spasm can make future births difficult, and the possibility of course exists that the unresolved conflicts which caused the vaginismus may be unconsciously transmitted to the woman's children.

Our capacity to become good mothers may also be seriously compromised when the forces which drive us are the powerful, unresolved fantasies about babies without sex (i.e., virgin births).[39]

Finally, while I've explained the reasons why AIH may not always be appropriate, I believe a woman should ultimately have the right to choose what she wishes to do with her body.

LIVING WITH VAGINISMUS

The presence of vaginismus can have a devastating effect on the quality of our lives. Unlike other female sexual problems (for example, lack of orgasm), vaginismus forbids both penetration and the ability to conceive, thereby striking at the very core of human creation: our ability to make new life. Vaginismus, therefore, is unique in that it cruelly combines the misery of a sexual problem with the anguish of childlessness.

> Vaginismus has affected my whole life, taken away all my confidence and turned me into a very solitary person. I feel totally inadequate and inferior.
>
> —Valerie

LOSS OF FEMININITY AND STATUS AS A WIFE

Vaginismus made me feel different from all other women. It placed my femininity in question because being a woman is so deeply connected with making love and making children, neither of which I was able to do.

> I felt a fraud. To others I appeared happily married and seemed to be doing the same things as my friends, but I never felt involved with them.
>
> —Sarah

I also felt a great lack of control in losing power over two major functions of female life: the ability to use my vagina sexually and the ability to reproduce. Because of my age and married state, I felt ashamed of my virginity. I hurt inside all the time, but the complexity of my emotions made me harsh and unsympathetic with myself.

> We thought of annulment but couldn't face the parental anger.
>
> —Jean

The validity of a heterosexual marriage in society is solely defined by whether or not it has been sexually consummated. In fact, the law places such importance on nonconsummation that a marriage can be annulled and any special qualities which might exist in such a union seemingly dismissed. In the eyes of society and the law the virginity of a wife invalidates her marriage, making her feel, as I did, that she and her partner are living a lie.

> I felt a total failure . . . I wasn't a whole woman because I couldn't have intercourse.
>
> —Sarah

EXCLUSION FROM THE SEXUAL AND FERTILE WORLD

Seeing pregnant women and women with children was a continual reminder of my exclusion from a sexually active world where women make love with their partners and bear children. Sex and pregnancy are ever-present and inescapable.

> As each of my friends became pregnant I felt quite devastated.
> I felt envious because their pregnancies became proof to me
> that they had actually done something I hadn't.
>
> —Sarah

Even a trip to the supermarket or a walk past stores selling maternity and baby clothes would produce intense feelings of envy directed toward the women around me, resulting in a deep depression. While I felt ashamed of my angry impulses, this merely reinforced my feelings of self-loathing. When I was at my lowest my childlessness, combined with the envy, anger and guilt, made me feel that my only escape from pain would be to end my life.

Being with married friends was also painful. It seemed to me that they were constantly talking about contraception or their sex lives and, if that wasn't bad enough, the wives appeared to be forever getting pregnant. This became proof to me of their fertility and their lovemaking, which my partner and I could not enjoy.

> I think the hardest and loneliest time for me was during my
> friends' pregnancies. I just wondered where my life was going
> to lead after that.
>
> —Sarah

Likewise, maintaining friendships with women, especially when they were pregnant, became increasingly difficult. I felt tormented by the images I had of their fecund bodies. Because they could have penetration I fantasized that they had magical holes or cavernous spaces where their vaginas were, and I felt a million miles away from them in terms of my physical size and mental growth.

Sadly for some of us, it's not even possible to enjoy friendships with women:

> I don't have girlfriends and don't get on with other women. My therapist thinks this has to do with my feeling inferior because I still feel less than a woman.
>
> —Jan

LACK OF PROFESSIONAL HELP AND UNDERSTANDING

Because vaginismus is such an intimate problem, we often believe we have to resolve it ourselves. This makes it hard for us even to begin to ask for professional help:

> I was far too frightened and embarrassed to go to my GP. He was always so brusque with me and overworked.
>
> —Sarah

Even if we seek professional help, the most appropriate treatment may not always be offered at the first consultation:

> My husband and I went to see about seven doctors before we finally got to the one who passed me on to the psychologist who actually treated me.
>
> —Jan

The pain of my vaginismus was worsened by the rejecting responses I received from doctors I first contacted. At best they were reassuring but ill-informed, telling me to "just relax, have some alcohol and it will pass." At worst their responses were cold and indifferent, such as "Pull yourself together." I blamed myself, my demands and my vaginismus for these responses, but it was only as I began to encounter other sufferers who had received identical responses that I learned to take these remarks less personally:

He told me to go and get drunk, let myself go and I'd be fine.

—Valerie

At his suggestion I tried getting drunk . . . a whole bottle of vodka. I was revoltingly sick with an appalling hangover . . . no use at all . . . They didn't understand me at the gyne-cological clinic either, and said I'd have to pull myself together.

—Jean

The power to heal vaginismus lies within the woman and in her ability to create a healing partnership with the doctor or therapist of her informed choice. In sharing these experiences, I am not accusing all doctors of being intentionally uncaring. However, I've noticed in reading other self-help books about women's health that the common solution to any problem has been the suggestion that a woman seek the help of a GP or another doctor or "expert." The writers rarely acknowledge or prepare the reader for the fact that it may not be that easy to find someone who is caring, skilled and understanding and who can help you on the first attempt.

I saw various doctors, sex therapists and hypnotherapists before I received the appropriate help.

—Valerie

There were only two doctors out of eight who helped me. The first gave me a manual which helped me see it wasn't just my inability to make love but rather I suffered from a definite condition. The second doctor referred me to the clinical psychologist.

—Jan

ISOLATION AND CONCEALMENT OF TRUTH

No one knows about it . . . I'm far too ashamed. I know I would have to emigrate if anyone ever found out.

—Valerie

Vaginismus is an invisible handicap. Looking at me, you would never know that I had the condition, and unless I tell people they never know. Because I was unable to allow my problem to be acknowledged, I didn't feel I was being authentic. In other words, I wasn't being true to myself or others. The very nature of vaginismus—the fact that it manifests in the most intimate part of my body—made me feel I had to struggle alone and manage for myself.

The pressure to behave as if everything is all right can eventually become unbearable:

> I seemed to be weeping for weeks on end . . . my husband wept too . . . but all the while pretending at work and to friends I was having a very torrid sex life.
>
> —Jean

Despite its invisibility, we still fear our vaginismus can somehow be sensed by others:

> It has made my life a very sad and lonely one, as I don't feel that I can mix . . . I feel that people will guess why I'm like I am.
>
> —Valerie

> I was frightened to open up in any way about myself in case people got to my deadly secret.
>
> —Sarah

ALIENATION FROM THE FAMILY

Perhaps the most difficult pain of all to cope with was the obvious concern (yet insidious pressure) I felt from my family and my husband's because of our childlessness. I wasn't able to explain my vaginismus, since I felt ashamed, feared rejection and believed nobody would understand.

I didn't once think of telling anyone. Even now that it's all sorted out I still wouldn't . . . I think I would have died rather than tell anyone.

—Sarah

Our childlessness was explained away as infertility. This led to my being swamped with well-meaning advice from family, friends and even strangers about one infertility treatment or another, which was just another terrible reminder that I wasn't being truthful with the people around me. This led to my feeling further isolated and believing that nobody knew the real me.

I think the worst part of having vaginismus is that you can't tell anyone . . . you feel so alone with it. It's not like having a moan to your friends about the sort of problems you can all have a natter about . . . it's a taboo subject.

—Helen

I hate to think there are lots of other people living like this. There seems to be a "club" for most other problems, but this just isn't the sort of problem you can bring up for fear of being made fun of.

—Valerie

In the midst of my loneliness and isolation, I longed to unburden myself to my mother. But what would she say? How would she react? I felt too embarrassed to make such an intimate confession. My fear of her disgust and rejection reflected my own judgmental attitude toward myself: my inability to tell my mother had far more to do with me than with her. As I discovered when I finally told my parents, my fears and fantasies about how they would respond bore little relation to their actual response, which was one of love and understanding, combined with the lament, "If only you'd told us before . . . we could have helped you."

Sometimes, however, the response is not the one we hoped for:

At twenty I tried to tell [Mother], but she was angry with
me and couldn't understand. All the years she'd said "never
let a man touch you there" . . . and I hadn't . . . and when
at last it was allowed, I couldn't.

—Jean

Because of increased media coverage about test-tube babies
and surrogate mothers, people are more aware of the effects
of infertility and the plight of infertile couples. The stress of
being childless can be so great that it has reportedly led to
divorce and, in some cases, suicide. If childlessness is stressful
in itself, imagine the additional stress when it results from,
and is combined with, the inability to make love.

CAN VAGINISMUS BE TREATED?

Vaginismus is distressing, but it can be relieved, and there's
a high chance of success.

—Dr. Paul Brown

Sometimes you can reach success quite quickly. I've had these
lovely cases where women are transformed in about two vis-
its. They come back and they look different. Sometimes you
can hardly recognize a woman who comes into the room
because she suddenly belongs to herself.

—Dr. Katharine Draper

Vaginismus can be successfully treated, and often is. However, such success may depend on the woman's ability to find
a sensitive, skilled therapist as well as to find the strength
and commitment within herself to engage in such a process.

It is important to state that vaginismus can be treated.
Before I sought help, and even at times during therapy, I had
a deep conviction that it was untreatable.

I never knew that doctors could refer you to people who could
help. I never had the feeling that vaginismus could be treated.

—Jan

The fear that vaginismus is too big a problem to be treatable originates in infancy, when a baby might feel her problems and emotions are too overwhelming and daunting for her to deal with. Again, noticing the connection between today's feelings and my past was an important step in the healing process for me.

Vaginismus can be treated by a range of methods, most commonly behavioral and sexual therapies, psychotherapy, or a combination. Vaginismus is reported to respond very well, and the prognosis is generally excellent for sufferers. As confirmed by Sarrel, Sarrel and Nadelson, it is a rare case of vaginismus which cannot be treated. When failure occurs, it is usually due to premature termination or the presence of other problems, in either the woman or her partner.[40] (I will discuss treatment methods in Chapter Five.)

To summarize: vaginismus is not rare. Though for a long time it was not fully recognized, it has always existed, and once appropriate help is sought the outcome is generally positive.

Chapter 3

WHAT CAUSES VAGINISMUS?

There are as many different reasons for vaginismus as there are different women. I always see it never being *one* thing that causes anything. It's several factors gradually merging together, and a whole cluster of additional factors that come around that, and then a further cluster of factors around that.

—Jill Curtis, psychotherapist

NOT ONE PARTICULAR EVENT OR CAUSE

For the majority of women who suffer from vaginismus, the causes can be identified with a stage or stages in psychological development from which we were unable to move on. If we get stuck at a phase in development, the growth necessary to carry us on to genital maturity may not take place. However, it is rarely possible to trace the causes to one particular incident. Usually, nothing specific has taken place, so few of us can blame vaginismus on a particular trauma or event. Not being able to pinpoint a definitive cause of an emotional problem may be one reason that psychotherapy is frequently dismissed as ineffective.

If one specific cause cannot be found, the condition only becomes more frustrating and puzzling for the sufferer. That may be the reason we ask ourselves, "Why have I got vaginismus? How did it happen? Is it my fault? If not mine, whose?" I have agonized over these questions, and I suspect that other women have, too. The truth is, it is nobody's fault that we have vaginal spasm:

> Women need to somehow take a compassionate stance toward themselves. This spasm is an attempt to protect themselves from something, but what exactly we don't know. The way that she is going to change it is to try and understand what it means for her, how it serves her and how she might express whatever conflict it expresses more directly.
> —Susie Orbach, psychotherapist

It is unfortunate that when looking for the causes of problems, all too often we are tempted to fall into the trap of "Who's to blame?" Blame has no place when one is looking at the origins of vaginismus or indeed of any emotional difficulty. It might be more helpful to begin by asking, "What is the spasm protecting me from?" Asking this can open the doors to understanding how and why we developed vaginismus, rather than attempting to blame ourselves or others. It also allows us to make contact with our power, creativity, love and responsibility, all of which are necessary in resolving problems.

Highly Individual Causes

A wide variety of factors may play a role in the causes, as they did in my case, and no single pattern emerges as definitive. Each cause has unique components for each woman which may only become apparent as therapy progresses. What is quite clear is that psychological factors play a far greater part than physical factors.

> The obvious causes to look for are actual trauma, where something unpleasant has happened about the vagina (a learned experience), or where the woman has got cultural condition-

ing that says sex is bad (an attitudinal experience), or she may have a much deeper unconscious basis connected with her own sexuality as a woman.

> —Dr. Paul Brown, consulting clinical psychologist

There could be a trigger incident at adolescence . . . but the makings of a personality happen very early on.

> —Susie Orbach

Many practitioners I spoke with agree that it is very hard to say what causes vaginismus. For example, the issues which often underlie the condition (fear of intimacy and loss of control, as well as low self-esteem) are not exclusive to the woman who suffers from vaginismus. There may be little difference between the histories of a woman who suffers from vaginismus and one who does not.

While a combination of influences may be common, the incidence of one or more does not automatically lead to vaginismus, but suggests that other factors may also be involved. Many women with similar backgrounds (sisters or women who have experienced similar or more severe traumas) do not develop vaginismus:

> Working psychoanalytically, I am trying to put together the pieces in a jigsaw that are so complex for each individual woman. I might even see a patient and think, "Why doesn't she have vaginismus with this kind of history?", but [she] clearly doesn't. The causes of vaginismus will be so individual, but there are general themes: women's feelings of unentitlement, the fact we're brought up to be terrified of our bodies and sexuality, that our bodies aren't for us, they're for somebody else.
>
> —Susie Orbach

OUR PAST SHAPES OUR PRESENT

Even if it is not always intentional, most professions find themselves shrouded in mystery, and psychoanalysis is no exception. Yet when we have the opportunity to understand the workings of a profession we are often amazed to see how much of it is based on common sense. You may be surprised to recognize personal experiences in this section. You might even think to yourself, "Oh, so that's why I feel this way . . ." An understanding of our emotional life may trigger greater understanding of the relationship between early psychological development and our vaginismus, and this recognition of the connection between past and present can be a key to resolution.

Psychological factors tend to fall into three main categories:[1]

1. Developmental (by far the most common)
   - emotional stress occurring at a sensitive period of development leading to arrest of psychological growth
   - upbringing invested with guilt, shame and misinformation about sex; strict religious taboos
2. Traumatic
   - rape
   - female genital mutilation
   - childhood sexual abuse
   - clumsy or brutal first-time sex
   - painful vaginal examinations
3. Relational:
   - inadequate foreplay contributing to lack of arousal
   - fear of being overheard or interrupted during sex
   - partner's impotence or sexual ineptitude
   - negative attitudes and feelings toward a lover
   - conflict and stress in a relationship
   - feeling dominated and oppressed by men

DEVELOPMENTAL FACTORS

To simplify somewhat, I think that in most cases vaginismus is a lack or disturbance of a good relationship with mother.
                                                                —Frances

Incredibly, it was in going back to my infancy★ that most of the causes of my vaginismus were identified. Early psychological development is critical and shapes adult behavior. Some of the origins of vaginismus can be traced to a disturbance in the relationship between mother and infant; others to a reaction a child has to infantile fantasies dating from the first four years of her life.[2] Although the psychological traumas and anxieties inherent in my early growth are part of universal human experience, the effects on me were unique. It was not simply any events which caused my vaginismus, but rather the ways in which I perceived these incidents. In fact, many themes outlined here, though specific to vaginismus, are also evident in the origins of other emotional and sexual problems.

While much of the following is based on psychoanalytic theory, I have not simply extracted it from published information. Instead I have combined it with the discoveries I made along the journey I undertook with my therapist. We re-created the baby that I was.

THE BEGINNINGS

Imagine life in the womb: a place where hunger, thirst, cold and separation do not exist. Then we are born, and suddenly have to adapt to gravity and temperature, sounds and smells, hunger and other needs. To protect a baby from a premature sense of separation, there should be as much continuity as possible from uterus to outside world. The umbilical cord should be cut when it has stopped pulsating, and the baby should be placed immediately either on the mother's body or in her arms. The mother needs to introduce the world to her child in gradual stages, and only when the baby is ready

★ A detailed description of the complex processes relating to early psychological development is beyond the scope of this book. I have therefore attempted to abstract only aspects of special relevance to vaginismus. At the back of this book are some readings which you may find useful.

to cope with the reality and grief of separation from the mother.[3]

In the early weeks a baby's life is one of pure sensation: being held and fed, changed, stroked and bathed. Early physical contact plays an essential role in the origins of vaginismus. The mother needs to relate to her baby as an individual and not deny the baby's individuality. The mother needs to make her baby aware that although the mother adores her, the child is nevertheless separate, with a life of her own. This frees the baby to explore and seek to have her own needs met. We are talking here about the creation of boundaries, a central issue in the psychological makeup of vaginismic women.

A mother who is struggling with her own sense of identity and her own legacy of inadequate mothering will be unable to allow her baby separation (often referred to by psychoanalysts as individuation). The mother's need to "own" her baby and see her purely as an extension of herself can feel to the baby like an invasion, an impingement on her developing sense of self. Inevitably, though, the mother comes to realize that her baby has her own identity apart from the mother, and this comes as a shock. Unconsciously the mother feels outraged and disillusioned, and her anger and pain can lead to an inadequate response to the child.

A lack of boundaries can lead to feelings of confusion: the baby does not know where she ends and where her mother begins, making her feel unintegrated, as though her inner world is splitting. The problems of separation, impingement and merger—all of which the baby feels as a loss of self and threatened annihilation—force the baby to create the only boundary she can be certain about: her body, her vagina. Vaginismus becomes the protection the baby seeks from perceived merger with or invasion by the mother and later by others. (Boundary issues are also discussed in the section of this chapter called "Psychological Separation from Parents," page 66; "Creating a Defensive Boundary," page 95; and "Self-Examination/Exploration," page 210.)

BABY'S PERCEPTIONS

Positive experiences in infancy can work toward healthy emotional development, with consistency in love and care creating a sense of well-being and promoting a positive self-image and self-love. My ability to take in good things from my parents and enjoy such feelings depended not only on real, but also on perceived events during my early development. I now realize that frustrating or upsetting experiences in my infancy were not always caused by inadequate care or attention. When I was a baby, my hunger, pain and discomfort, even if they lasted only two or three minutes, were distressing. My upset did not necessarily signify my mother's intentional withholding or willful lack of care, but to be a baby and to feel unhappy with Mother was to be angry with my whole world. My mother's presence was felt to be most powerful in my life, and I perceived myself as a helpless recipient of good or bad experiences—a kind of emotional puppet on a string. If mothers have difficulty in connecting with and relating to their babies because of their own psychology and social conditioning, the absence of connection may make the process of separation between the two of them more troublesome.[4]

But how did my anxieties and perceptions become real to me? This has to do with my unconscious, the contents of which consist mainly of unfinished business and other related matters from childhood, tensions which never become conscious, or which perhaps once were and have been repressed. An imagining or fantasy may be just as real to a baby's unconscious as an actual experience. Many of my mental images of people or events have little connection with reality, and yet are just as influential on my behavior as if they did. For example, a "good" internal image of my mother may have been based on memories or fantasies of what she was like.[5]

GOOD MOTHER, BAD MOTHER

Theories developed since Freud suggested that when the person on whom a baby relies for growth and love (usually the mother) is unable to respond consistently or satisfactorily to the baby's needs, the infant creates a world of internal relationships ("internal object relations") to cope with the disappointments and difficulties she experiences.[6] This process is called introjection. As a baby, I internalized images of important emotional figures (my parents); thus, my internalized image of my mother may have had far more to do with my unreal desires and fears about her than the way in which she actually felt or behaved toward me. However, the emotions these fantasies aroused were real.

Because my mother was still needed for my survival, I felt unable to condemn her and consequently took into my developing psychology the idea that it was not her responses that were inadequate or inappropriate but rather my selfish, insatiable, devouring, bad (and even loving) needs that were the cause of all my problems.* I thus admonished myself and attempted to bury my needs, creating a fantasy world in which badly experienced aspects of my mother ("bad object") were reconstructed. (See the section of Chapter Five called "Linda's Treatment," page 154.) This bad object became split into two images: one part became my teasing, powerful, much-needed mother and the other my rejecting, nasty, hateful mother. The overwhelming presence of persecutory fantasies forced me to develop what is called a false self, that is, one which is devoid of needs and shows itself to be undemanding, carefree and contented.

My unnurtured true self had been separated and repressed.[7] Sufficiently secure development was consequently thwarted

---

* The discovery I made in analysis was the fact that it was not simply that my needs made me ashamed, but also that my *love* was destructive. If needs remain unmet and the baby feels hateful, she believes her love *and* her hate are the cause of her unhappiness.

and the growth required to take me on to the next stage could not be completed. Most of us manage to unknowingly work through these emotions, but when fantasies about my power and destructiveness became real to me, problems began to occur.

PSYCHOLOGICAL SEPARATION FROM PARENTS

Most analysts agree that the roots of all sexual and emotional problems are unresolved conflicts occurring at specific stages in childhood. They call all repressed childhood experiences and accompanying emotions complexes, the most important of which is widely recognized as the Oedipus complex.[8] This was the stage in my development, between the ages of four and five, when I experienced feelings of natural eroticism toward my father.

The potential for a child to break away psychologically from her mother and father and enter the adult world to seek a sexual partner of her own will depend very much on the outcome of this stage of development. Because the origins of vaginismus are often related to early, intense, unconscious envy and rivalry of mother's ability to give father things we cannot, the Oedipal stage is of great significance in the development of vaginismus.* (This aspect is further described in "Linda's Treatment" in Chapter Five.)

WHEN REAL EVENTS BECOME DISTORTED

Psychoanalysis has shown us that it is quite normal for a developing girl to have a rich and varied fantasy life, depending on her abilities, talents, and intelligence. Whether a fantasy is pleasant or sadistic will depend on the psychological

---

* Many analysts after Freud regard the period when the baby is totally dependent, not the Oedipal phase, as the stage of development when psychological problems may occur.

age of a child, and these fantasies seemed to play an important role when I was being analyzed.[9]

My own therapy, and the psychoanalytic literature, support the notion that little girls fear as well as desire penetration. However, Sarrel, Sarrel and Nadelson cite an alternative suggestion that all human beings are "instinctively" afraid of bodily penetration of any sort. It therefore makes sense to assume that negative experiences may increase penetration anxiety.[10]

Whereas "fantasies" are conscious, "fantasies" are unconscious imaginings. They control our thoughts, emotions and behavior, as well as the assumptions we make about ourselves. A fantasy may have occurred whereby as a baby I feared injury by a penis to my vagina, leading to expectation of painful intercourse. This fantasy may have been the result of my accidentally seeing my parents making love (called the primal scene), resulting in my imagining and distorting activities around me.★ Such distorted interpretations of the sexual act or my parents' relationship may have damaged or arrested my essential psychological growth. This fantasy produced inner feelings of guilt, envy and unlovability, manifesting themselves in vaginismus and effectively preventing love and intimacy from entering me later on.

DESIRING AND FEARING THE PENIS
AT THE SAME TIME

When a girl develops emotionally, her vagina plays a more important role in her fantasies.[11] She may have magical ideas about what the penis does to the mother's body. The penis's disappearance into the mother during sex becomes the mother's snatching away of the penis. In other words, I may have

★ The primal scene is not only the witnessing of parental intercourse, but describes any event during which a baby perceives or imagines an exciting, tantalizing but excluding relationship between her parents.

felt so angry that I had no penis that I unconsciously wished to castrate men in revenge for my own castration. This fantasy is called the castration complex, and Freud claimed it is universal to the development of girls. It is particularly mentioned in psychoanalytic writings as a prototype in explaining vaginismus.

So, for me as a baby the penis was both the desired organ, evoking envy, and the feared organ, evoking anxiety that it would damage my vagina. In the past, analysts always presumed that vaginismus is a woman's unconscious wish to snatch away the penis and that unresolved penis envy is likely to result in vaginismus in later life. However, though practitioners can confirm these concepts, they should not be taken as the general rule. Clinical experience does not confirm the theory that all sufferers have intense penis envy.★ One doctor observes that while some women with vaginismus feel anger toward their lovers, just as many show no signs of hostility and are relieved and elated when able to accept penetration and give pleasure.[12]

Penis envy is not the only infantile fantasy which can give rise to vaginismus, and indeed not all therapists work within the Freudian framework of such theories:

> I don't see genital relations as an expression of adulthood. I would be looking at what vaginismus means in terms of the "internal object relations." That is, how the woman has translated the world of people into an internal world and how that world satisfies or doesn't satisfy her. I don't mean at only a sexual level, but rather how it meets her needs for love and contact.
>
> —Susie Orbach

★ Orthodox Freudians and writers on vaginismus believe the condition to be the result of a castration fantasy. While this may play a role in the development of some women, I noted that it did not emerge in the therapies of the women I interviewed, nor indeed in my own.

It may help to remember that Freud's theories about feminine psychology were developed by a Victorian man. The penis should be seen not simply as a physical organ but also as what it represents symbolically for the baby, that is, how she has translated the world of people into a world of objects such as penis, breast, and so on. As a symbol of aggression, for example, the penis might stand for the freedom to be, to force one's way, to get what one wants.[13] Viewed in this way, envy of the penis may mean anger and envy connected with much wider issues, not necessarily related to men. (These issues are discussed further in the section of this chapter called "Women in Society," page 90.)

A GIRL'S SUSCEPTIBILITY TO VAGINISMUS

Most child psychologists find that the fantasies I have described also occur in emotionally and physically normal girls. If such fantasies are common to us all, why does vaginismus appear only in certain women? It may be that some girls have a predisposition* toward a particular emotional condition.

If a girl's personality (ego) has strong natural defenses it can help her overcome sexual fears. However, important hereditary factors may have played a part in determining my emotional development and strength, predisposing me to a certain defense mechanism. It is known, for example, that some defense reflexes are transmitted between members of one family, explaining why some people have a special disposition to isolation or depression. I had an innate tendency to repression, forcing me to express emotional pain through

---

* We must be careful when using such terms as "predisposition," "hereditary factors" and "susceptibility," because normally these imply some relation to biological symptoms or traits present since birth. However, with regard to vaginismus such meanings are irrelevant because what counts is the attitudes of a girl's parents, other adults and contemporaries toward her sexuality. Therefore, when I refer to predisposition and hereditary factors it is to suggest that vaginismus evolves from a combination of past and present circumstances. It is not something organic.

my body—through vaginismus.[14] Because of these hereditary factors I probably became fixed at a phase in development which the nonvaginismic woman has been able to pass through unknowingly.

A defense is a creative mechanism meant to protect me psychologically. It is an adaptation which has arisen out of fear and upset, operating in self-destructive as well as self-protective ways. Vaginismus attempts to keep out rejections and disappointments, but can also simultaneously prevent nourishment and love from coming in. The hidden part of my psyche has developed vaginismus to protect me from anticipated pain and disappointment[15] and, in so doing, paradoxically prevents me from feeling loved.

STRESS IN A SENSITIVE PHASE OF DEVELOPMENT

It is likely that I failed to overcome a normal stressful situation at a sensitive phase of development, possibly due to hereditary factors. Stressful situations (real or imagined) which occur during the infantile and Oedipal phases of development can contribute to the onset of vaginismus. As a child I returned (regressed) to an earlier stage in which my personality had been less troubled. I thus took refuge in the stage of emotional growth where magical thinking about my body and my vagina was typical.[16]

OWNERSHIP OF ONE'S VAGINA

> There seems to be an inability in the woman with vaginismus to acquire an ease of genital activity.
>
> —Jill Curtis

The path from girlhood to maturity is never an easy one, and the leap from being a little girl to being an adult is a major psychological hurdle.

When I was small I did not "own" my body, in the sense

that I needed my mother to feed me, bathe me, dress me and even think for me. Depending on our gender, Mother will choose whether our outfit is to be pink or blue. Perhaps we can recall the time when we suddenly knew we had to take care of our own bodies; this might have been when Mother told us to wash our own necks, or perhaps it was the time when she no longer straightened our stockings or did our hair. In this sequence of unconscious events, the last piece of her body to be psychologically handed over to a girl is her vagina. In a way, it symbolizes the final piece of her childhood.

Because of unconscious prohibitions transmitted from my parents, I may have felt unable to make this leap to owning my genitals with ease. If I felt I must remain an emotionally obedient daughter, I could not then seek my own lover; the ties to my parents caused me to doubt the rightness of my needs and desires. I could not see myself as lover or wife, but merely as their little girl.

This ability to own one's vagina marks womanhood in psychosexual terms. If the path to emotional maturity is such that a girl feels guilty at no longer being the dutiful daughter, she may be too anxious to leave childhood. In a psychological sense I remained that child whose vagina did not yet belong to me to enjoy, own or use without parental permission.

THE ADULT AS MODEL

In order to aspire to maturity and acquire her own sexuality, a girl needs not only to psychologically own her vagina, but also to admire and envy the adults around her enough to wish to be like them, emulate them, and finally join their world.

However, if the gap between the girl's admiration and wish to be like the adults becomes too wide (because of over-whelming envy, persecutory fantasies or a hostile environment), the necessary psychological growth cannot take place. Biologically I reached adulthood, but I was never able to psychologically acquire my vaginal maturity; my jealousy and envy of adults were too overwhelming.

WHEN COMMUNICATIONS ARE UNINTENTIONALLY NEGATIVE

Early perceptions of my parents may also have been crucial, since their characters and personalities largely determined the attitudes which existed in my home. In this way parents may consciously or unconsciously communicate their fears and anxieties:

> I suppose the belief that I took on board was that little girls don't have sex . . . so actually I'm being "good" at the moment because I'm not having sex.
>
> —Jan

Because such messages tend to be more intensely transmitted to firstborn or only children, many women with vaginismus, like me, are either the eldest in the family, the only daughter or the only child.

My mother's feelings about her body and sexuality strongly influenced how I came to feel. If a mother unconsciously stifles a girl's natural curiosity about her body, it may instill the sense that the vagina is forbidden, mysterious and unwholesome territory. It should be understood that much of this negative conditioning, heavily influenced by the mother's psychology and social factors, takes place in a gentle and well-intentioned way, rarely meant to harm or instill fear. I recall my mother telling me she disliked and couldn't insert tampons. Though this was never meant to frighten me, it nevertheless resulted in negative feelings, compounding my already developing fear about inserting anything into my vagina.

Studies confirm that girls who try repeatedly to insert a tampon but continue to fail despite very determined efforts or the assistance of someone else tend to believe that they are not constructed normally. Such an early experience of vaginismus is in response to the threat of penetration, and this kind of difficulty with a tampon is frequently elicited in the histories taken from vaginismic women.[17]

> A fairly common thing that vaginismic women report is that they got stuck when they first tried to use tampons. The girl who gains confidence to do this and manages it has a tremendous boost to her confidence. For the girl who doesn't manage it, it's devastating because her fantasy is that she's either different from her friends or that she's too small.
> —Dr. Anne Mathieson, medical hypnotherapist

Although it is usually only a single incident, it often has a lasting effect, perhaps because it is in the context of a new experience.[18]

Specialists express a diversity of opinions as to the causes of vaginismus that may be related to communications in the family home. Some report that vaginismus is the result of a sexually repressed upbringing, but just as many refute this, stating that women who have had repressed childhoods are more likely to be generally sexually unresponsive and anorgasmic than to develop vaginismus. Women who have vaginismus, on the other hand, are often found to be very sexual, not inhibited as might be expected if their backgrounds had been repressive.

THE LANGUAGE OF THE VAGINA

The link between my development and my subsequent fantasies was crucial to the understanding and treatment of my vaginismus, because the unconscious anxieties I had developed, for whatever reasons, were directly related to the onset of vaginismus. A specific fantasy a woman expresses can often be the key to understanding and treating the condition.[19] When I say something about my vagina, I may be saying something similar about my innermost fears and desires, giving clues to the origins of vaginismus. In Chapter Five we will see how often women make the same claims about their feelings: they fear the vagina is too small, they claim to be ignorant about sex and their bodies, they fear intercourse will be painful, they fear they will be damaged. These are themes we express over and over again.

But why, you may ask, are we expressing how we feel in this particular way? Perhaps if there is a part of us that feels isolated, unloved, hidden, rejected, abandoned and infantile, yet remains unknown to us, this is the only way we can express such emotions:

- "My vagina is too small." Are we really saying that the adult in us is too small? Perhaps our wants, needs and unnurtured selves make us feel too small, too young, too undeveloped and too vulnerable.

- "My vagina is a dark and dirty place." Are we really saying that the sexy sides of our natures, or our emotional needs and desires, are dark, dirty, need cleaning up or merit apology?

- "I wasn't told about sex. I knew my parents did it but I never felt I could." Are we really saying that we need our parents' blessing, encouragement and permission to have desires and needs?

- "Intercourse will be painful; I'll be damaged and torn." Are we really saying that our desires for love and intimacy are also dangerous, damaging and overwhelming and need controlling?

- "The thought of being penetrated makes me want to retch." Are we really saying that our needs and desires are too much for us to digest, that it's too soon to take them inside us, that we aren't ready?

We can see that vaginismus is very much a metaphor for our innermost fears and feelings about our needs and desires. However, none of us will use her body unconsciously to express the same thing, nor do we share the same language:

> There are common themes in women's psychology about being fearful of intimacy, feeling unentitled to love. But what the particulars are for each woman will be totally individual.
> —Susie Orbach

The developmental aspects demonstrate that vaginismus is not necessarily the result of willfully inadequate care or love from parents. It has far more to do with the complex combination of our inherent predisposition, our psychological development, our personality, the personalities of our caregivers and their social conditioning, and our perceptions.

Dr. Robina Thexton of London's Institute of Psychosexual Medicine further highlights this last point:

> It's the girl's perceptions of her family and relationships rather than what they do. Sometimes it can be the most unexpected women who have vaginismus in that they appear to have had healthy, happy mothers, lovely opportunities and loving relationships . . . and surprisingly find they have this problem.

TRAUMATIC FACTORS

A trauma is a powerful incident or psychological shock which can sometimes have a lasting effect upon well-being.

Though not cited as a major cause of vaginismus, trauma may have played a part in its onset in some women.

RAPE

> I was first raped at sixteen . . . but I don't know whether I
> had vaginismus before that.
>
> —Jan

> I've treated women who had great problems after rape, so
> vaginismus can definitely develop after this.
>
> —Dr. Robina Thexton

Other doctors have confirmed that vaginismus can develop
in a woman previously not suffering from the condition after
a trauma such as rape. In addition, if rape is committed on
a sexually immature girl, the effects can be so disturbing that
her psychosexual makeup may be damaged.

CHILDHOOD SEXUAL ABUSE

Vaginismus as a consequence of childhood sexual abuse is
rarely mentioned in current medical literature. Perhaps its
absence is a reflection that as a general issue child abuse has
been greatly suppressed. Only in more recent years has the
issue been more openly discussed. Doctors and therapists
confirm that while only a small number of sufferers from
vaginismus have been sexually abused as children, such abuse
can nevertheless be a cause.

> We have to be careful and say that not all women who have
> vaginismus have been sexually abused. However, many of
> the women we work with have developed a spasm as a result
> of their being sexually abused as a child.
>
> —Richard Johnson, Director,
> Incest Crisis Line,
> Northolt, Middlesex, England

It is suggested that professionals should inquire carefully
about beatings, inappropriate or frightening sexual advances,

actual molestation or rape. Where these experiences involved vaginal (or anal) penetration by finger, object or penis, the sensitizing effect is that much greater.[20]

BRUTAL FIRST–TIME SEX

Brutal or painful early sexual experience, perhaps with a clumsy or insensitive lover, may also set the stage for vaginismus:

> One woman had a rather brutal first husband, after which she couldn't make love the second time around and came for help.
>
> —Dr. Robina Thexton

PAINFUL VAGINAL EXAMINATIONS

Sometimes the causes of vaginismus are said to be iatrogenic, meaning that the symptom has been aggravated or even induced as the result of a doctor's words or actions:

> Of the three women I've seen today, two have been very badly hurt by a previous cervical smear and examination which has compounded the problem for them.
>
> —Dr. Robina Thexton

Traumatic pelvic examinations are cited as being contributing factors to, if not a sole cause of vaginismus. Dr. Katharine Draper comments with dismay about such examinations:

> I think doctors have quite a lot to answer for in the area of vaginismus. In the study that we [the Institute of Psychosexual Medicine] did, we asked women if they'd had a previous traumatic penetrative experience, not just vaginal but also rectal. A lot of dental treatment can also be transferred down to this part of the body. The number of women we met who'd had things said to them by doctors like "You're a bit small . . . you'll have trouble when you get married" . . . and then the fear grows and grows.

In the same way, nurse-therapist Barbara Lamb registers her concern and surprise at the insensitivity of some procedures:

> I feel doctors in VD clinics must not always assume the woman has been sexually active. One sufferer had not had proper penetration, but was a contact with a man who was found to have gonorrhea. She went along to a clinic where they carried out lengthy tests while she was still a virgin. It was so traumatic that it took two years for us to work through together.

One doctor I saw in the hope that he could help me though I was unable to tell him my real problem, attempted to introduce his finger into my vagina, as I had complained of "swelling down there." On seeing my difficulty, he angrily pried my legs apart and admonished me for being so childish. He then added, "As a married woman, you really ought to know better." Why was this doctor totally unable to recognize vaginismus in a woman so obviously vaginismic as me?

While such an experience did not cause my vaginismus, the trauma of being subjected to a brutal examination, both verbally and physically, merely reinforced my fears about telling anyone or allowing anyone inside. How can we prevent iatrogenic vaginismus? One way is to point out to doctors and nurses, ideally during training, that vaginismus can actually be induced by a rough physical examination or an insensitive approach. Another is to suggest that when conducting a vaginal examination the use of the word "small" should be avoided.

FEMALE GENITAL MUTILATION★

Removing sensitive parts of the female genitalia in the form of clitoridectomy is practiced in many parts of the world, commonly among Muslim groups in Australia, Philippines, Malaysia, Pakistan, Indonesia, United Arab Emirates, South and North Yemen, Bahrain and Oman. In Africa, not a single country is spared this practice, but it is not practiced in Iraq, Syria, and Tunisia. Its origins are unclear, and although believed to have a religious basis it is not practiced in Saudia Arabia, the heart of Islam, nor is it mentioned in the Koran or Old Testament. It is carried out as part of the initiation in the transition from childhood to womanhood.

As described in Chapter Two (pages 20–21), this practice was done in nineteenth-century Europe to cure women of nymphomania and hysteria. As a form of controling her resistance and "rebelliousness" J.P. was mutilated by her physician to *cure* her vaginismus, but in reality vaginismus (including psychological trauma and infertility) can develop *after* mutilating surgery.

Female genital mutilation has recently reemerged in the United States and Europe where large numbers of immigrants from Africa and Asia have brought with them this practice. Clitoridectomy is banned in Britain, France, Sudan, and Sweden, although it continues underground. However, because there is no government health service in the United States no federal law can be enforced. Attempts continue to be made to document the existence of clitoridectomy in order to make it illegal, and it is hoped that since Canada has a national health service it may be easier to implement legislation there first. International black health workers believe the only effective way to ban this procedure is through reeducational programs and highlighting the harm which arises

★ Note: Thanks to the following for help with this section: Fran Hosken, Editor, Women's International Network News (Lexington, MA) and Shamis Dirir Shur, Black Women's Health Action Project (London, England).

following clitoridectomy: Because of this, and because I believe clitoridectomy should not be isolated from other women's health issues, including vaginismus, I have included it in this book.

OUR BIRTH EXPERIENCE

Not so long ago it was believed that the unborn child had no feelings or thoughts in its mother's womb, and that it only began to feel and think once it was a few weeks old. However, much more is now known about a baby's emotional life and the effects birth can have on its development. This might seem far-fetched, but if we consider that trauma in early childhood can affect us, why not something even earlier such as birth trauma?

In 1966 a French obstetrician, Frederick Leboyer, announced to a mostly skeptical medical world that he was convinced the emotional environment of birth had profound and lifelong effects on a person. In 1974 his book *Birth Without Violence* laid the groundwork for a new awareness and sensitivity surrounding both the mother's and the baby's birth experience. Leboyer demonstrated that the quieter and gentler a birth was, the closer and better adjusted the baby and its mother would be. He also claimed that his "naturally" delivered babies fared better and were more successful in later life.

> One of the causes of vaginismus can be birth traumas, which women sometimes go back to in hypnosis. You see, the first thing we ever learn about the vagina is going through mother's, and if that's a truly terrifying experience a woman may be left with the feeling that the vagina is a very dangerous place.
>
> —Dr. Anne Mathieson

It does not automatically follow that a long, arduous labor will produce vaginismus, because generally no one specific event will cause the condition. Re-birthing groups★ have shown us that our ideas and feelings about birth are very personal and have different connections for different women. Some women, for example, in talking about their births do not even speak of the vagina. One psychoanalyst said he uses a woman's imagery, fantasies or dreams about her birth as metaphors. For instance, if she imagines she was crushed and suffocated while in her mother's birth canal, the analyst would interpret this as the crushing, suffocating adult who would not let her have her own thoughts.

As yet there is no scientific evidence to prove or disprove the idea that birth trauma can contribute to emotional problems. However, I believe that any fantasies or imagery we have surrounding our births should be seen as enriching material which we and our therapists can work through. In this way, a woman's ideas about her entry into the world may be seen as yet another symbol and metaphor for her innermost fears and feelings.

Not all women who are exposed to trauma go on to develop vaginismus, and the occurrence of the condition in a woman previously not suffering seems to imply that she is somehow inherently predisposed to vaginismus. Perhaps the

★ Re-birthing is a simple, subtle and powerful breathing experience which puts a woman in touch with the pleasure of being alive and allows her to see her birth as an exciting, if frightening, irruption into the world. It is a cumulative process carried out over weeks and months. A woman lies down and breathes, usually in the presence of a trained Re-birther. For two hours or more she breathes ("conscious connected breathing") to help her release the panic of her first breath. In her breathing she reveals her basic attitudes toward life, and gradually her breath restores itself to the balance and harmony it would have known had it not been for the trauma of that first gasp. She can then experience breathing as a spontaneously cleansing rhythm rather than a fearful controlled machine. Positive effects have been to ease stressful situations by producing an intuitive sigh of release instead of breathtaking panic. Relationships may also become easier, safer and more committed, partly because they are so often controlled by unconscious fear of separation, caused by the memory of leaving mother's womb.[21]

tendency toward the condition remains dormant until triggered by the psychological effects of any event such as those outlined here.

RELATIONAL FACTORS

Causes of vaginismus are said to be relational when the onset of the condition is connected to a person or situation outside our control. For example, vaginismus may occur if a woman feels hostile toward her lover, or if the society or environment she lives in is intrusive and unsupporting. Here Dr. Robina Thexton illustrates the effects on a woman whose status has suddenly changed:

> Vaginismus is surprisingly common for people who have been living together, not married, and they have a wedding ceremony and then it starts. That always needs quite a lot of understanding.
>
> —Dr. Robina Thexton

PARTNERS

> Personally I feel that for some women the sexual partner can consciously or unconsciously provide the fuel to ignite her own deepest anxieties.
>
> —Lorna Guthrie, Jungian analyst

During my research I came across the opinion that a woman's lovers can either contribute to, cause or maintain her vaginismus. While partners in general are *not* the cause of women's vaginismus, their role is, nonetheless, significant.

If we think again about a little girl's development, a woman's vaginismus can be seen as an expression of a disturbed earlier relationship. In a way, vaginismus is an answer to or defense against an unresolved conflict with a key figure or figures in her life. However, her partner, lover or husband is not necessarily the key figure. She may transfer her conflicts with mother or father to *every* sexual partner, so that he (or she, in the case of a gay woman) then becomes an innocent player in her scenario.[22] This does not imply that a partner is never responsible for or connected to a woman's vaginismus. I do believe, though, that when looking at the partner we also have to take into account a woman's earlier relationships, which shape her choice of and feelings toward a current lover.

Can a Partner Cause Vaginismus and Can Vaginismus Cause Impotence?

Masters & Johnson report that vaginismus has a common association with primary impotence (no previous experience of erection) in the partner. They add that where primary impotence and vaginismus exist in a relationship it is often difficult to be sure whether the vaginismus existed before unsuccessful attempts at intercourse or whether it developed secondarily because of frustration at the man's impotence. In other words, can vaginismus cause impotence or can impotence cause vaginismus?[23]

> The man can become sensitized to the pain or difficulty so that he's frightened of penetrating eventually, but I think this happens out of the experience that he has . . . he doesn't actually bring that to the relationship.
>
> —Dr. Paul Brown

Masters & Johnson further report that if a man has a severe problem with premature ejaculation, his partner can develop vaginismus through repeated frustrated attempts at lovemaking.[24]

However, I do not believe that the male partner is likely to be the main cause of vaginismus, but rather that he may trigger causes lying dormant. In my experience, it was the *emotional* relationship between my husband and me which suffered most from the effects of my vaginismus.

Perhaps because Masters & Johnson only treated couples with sexual difficulties, they neglected to notice the effects vaginismus has on a relationship holistically, only concentrating on the way the condition affects couples sexually.

Can a Partner Maintain Vaginismus?

If a woman's lover has not caused her vaginismus, it has been suggested that he can maintain it. One therapist says that in most cases he sees the role of the husband as an important contributing factor in the maintenance, if not the cause, of vaginismus. He observes that some husbands unconsciously collude in maintaining their wife's vaginismus if they themselves have unresolved fears and anxieties about sex.[25] On the other hand,

> I haven't found this to be true. I've seen so many men help their partners with vaginismus that in no way are they colluding or maintaining her spasm.
>
> —Barbara Lamb

I would avoid making such generalizations about both the woman and her partner. While some men may unconsciously maintain vaginismus, perhaps by not encouraging the woman to seek help, just as many men do not.

Are Partners Alike in Personality

Again, a common view is that the man who chooses a woman with vaginismus is generally overly kind and gentle, passive and un-pushy, and usually has sexual problems of his own. This implies that in some way a man unconsciously recognizes and chooses a woman who can't allow penetration because he has unresolved conflicts about his sexuality.

The majority of doctors and therapists I met did not find this description of partners to be generally true. Psychologist

Paul Brown said that this is a particularly harmful generalization, since he sees plenty of marriages in which the man is passive and gentle but his partner does not have vaginismus. Dr. Brown also remarked that he does not believe vaginismus has anything to do with the degree of gentleness or kindness a husband demonstrates toward his wife:

> I remember one man where his wife's vaginismus caused tremendous stress but brought out the most loving side of him. However, I don't think it was because his wife had vaginismus; I think any distress that she had had would have caused the same loving response.

Another doctor told me that any sexual problems which from time to time cropped up in a relationship did so in a totally unexpected way in what she would call a normal pairing. In other words, she did not see any difference between the vaginismic women's partners and the other partners among her patients.

It's quite possible that a woman with vaginismus might unconsciously select a partner who is kind and tolerant, in the possibly mistaken hope that being so gentle, he will hurt her less during intercourse. However, this is not evidence that only weak, impotent, timid, unassertive men with hidden anxieties about their sexual role and potency are attracted to women who have vaginismus and therefore perpetuate their spasms. This view seems to depend on the assumption that any lover of a vaginismic woman who fails to conform to the stereotypical macho, extroverted, strong male image is somehow inherently attracted to that woman because she is unable to allow penetration. Disappointingly, it highlights the endurance of sexist images of "normal" male behavior. Again, I prefer not to generalize. While some partners are extremely kind and patient, just as many are not.

Supporting my view, one study concludes that there is striking diversity in the natures of vaginismic women and their partners and the relationships between them.[26]

The husbands cover a wide spectrum. They may be strong
or weak, confident or unsure, and some are angry and fed up
while others are protective and supportive.
—Dr. Anne Mathieson

However, it became apparent during my interviews that
the majority of sex therapists view the role of the partner of
the vaginismic woman as highly important. This probably
explains why traditional sex therapy generally accepts only
couples, not just the woman with vaginismus.

Time and time again we've seen that couples where the
woman has vaginismus have kind of chosen each other. Where
there is vaginismus in a relationship, the difficulty appears to
be all with the woman, but in reality there often is some
difficulty with her partner. This becomes apparent when he
starts experiencing erectile difficulties, although the woman
now is able to allow penetration.
—Alison Clegg, sex therapy training officer,
Relate Marriage Guidance

Findings confirm that in an unconsummated relationship
the partner's fear of causing pain combined with his own
anxieties about penetration may be important factors. If the
man is tentative and pulls back at the first sign of any anxiety
in the woman, they mutually reinforce one another's unconscious anxieties about intercourse.[27]
One sex therapist says he believes that a man has to be
somehow "different" if he continues in a relationship in which
vaginismus is uncured and continuing; another said that if a
man waits years and years without having intercourse, the
sufferer might need to ask herself why he is doing that.
The notion that there is a link between vaginismus and
male impotence does not explain why women in gay relationships also suffer from vaginismus. Since vaginismus is
not confined to the heterosexual woman, it follows that the
general assumptions made about her partner may be erroneous.

Emotional, Not Sexual Compatibility

Our lovers are generally suspected of having problems of impotence, sexual identity or low sex drive, but this assumption seems to arise out of a belief that the sexual problem of the woman is somehow mirrored in the man she is with. But is vaginismus truly about sexual receptivity? Isn't it more about emotional receptivity?

As psychotherapist Susie Orbach explains:

> The view that partners are impotent assumes that vaginismus doesn't happen in lesbian relationships and assumes it is only about penises. Whereas in fact to me it's so little about the penis and so much more about the woman and her capacity to feel loved.

Susie Orbach goes on to challenge the view that partners of sufferers belong to a certain type of personality, and the general assumption that these partners "fit" psychologically together. She says that although men are frightened of their own sexuality and may feel alarmed by vaginismus, she nevertheless believes the fit between couples is much more of an emotional one:

> One might, for instance, have a man who really wants to give love but doesn't know how to do it.

As if to confirm this, Frances describes the unconscious mutual attraction between her and a partner:

> I suspect that I tend to attract men at my own level of psychosexual development, who want to be given to, not to give.

We may all make unconscious choices about our partners, and there is no real way of knowing how those choices are affected by the fact that we have vaginismus. I do think that the choices we make regarding a sexual partner relate more to emotional than sexual compatibility. Again, Frances explains that she believes relating intimately begins at the breast, and describes how the problems of basic nurturing at the start of her life have unconsciously affected her emotional choice of men:

> What causes me much despair is that I think I seek a mother in a man. Unless he gives me all the love I've missed, I don't want to give anything.

Leonard Friedman found that although a high proportion of husbands in his study were described by wives as "kind, considerate and passive," these traits had no significance in predicting the outcomes of the relationships.[28] The same study also found that the husband's sexual potency showed no relationship to the outcome of therapy.[29]

It appears that neither the lover's personality, gender nor sexual abilities plays an important role, and I would only consider the personality of a partner to be significant if it was found that it had a detrimental effect on either the woman's well-being or the outcome of therapy.

The interplay between us and our lovers should be viewed simultaneously with other influences on our lives, but the roles they play should not be considered significant in either the causes or the outcome of treatment for vaginismus.

Examining the Partner's Role Without Blame

There is no doubt that we all have an instinctive knack for seeking out partners with emotional conflicts similar to our own; much has been written, for example, about the psychological fit between women and their alcoholic partners. Similarly, a woman with vaginismus may be unconsciously drawn to certain men because she believes they will not cause her pain. I call these subtle interactions the *dance* a couple has with each other.

Over the years the spasm-pain-failure syndrome resulted in my marriage's coming to resemble a fraternal coupling. Like Hansel and Gretel, my husband and I were devoted yet could not be lovers. The dance with my partner revolved around the fact that he seemed nonthreatening to me. Later, he revealed an excessive need to suppress his feelings of anger and aggression. My vaginismus may have fallen in with his penetration-equals–pain anxiety, which was triggered by our painful attempts at intercourse. Naturally sex should be tender, but aggression and anger are important aspects of lovemaking. A man who fears he may hurt his wife or lover—because of repeated failures—and who also has problems expressing anger may unconsciously encourage his partner to protect his vulnerabilities, since society says that men are not supposed to feel frightened. He won't push her and she won't push him. Women have told me that during treatment they came to feel disappointed with their partner's gentleness, since his "pushiness" was now needed to resolve her vaginismus.

Vaginismus may also sometimes conceal underlying marital problems, so that the spasm becomes a way of clinging to a relationship that works neither emotionally nor physically. Neither partner can accept the pain, grief and loss of the truth that their marriage is over. In speaking with women and in examining current literature, I have found that many of the observations and conclusions made about our partners have been felt by us as criticisms. In the light of this, I hope the interactions between a woman and her partner may be viewed by doctors and therapists in a more compassionate and nonjudgmental way.

To my knowledge no literature exists, written by a partner, which describes the effects vaginismus can have on his sexual identity and emotional well-being. These issues need to be further explored and understood, but men will only come forward if the atmosphere in which such topics are discussed is open, receptive and loving. (For more on this subject, see the section called "Vaginismic Women's Group with Parallel Partners Group" in Chapter Five, page 201.)

WOMEN IN SOCIETY

"Relational causes" does not just mean the relationship between a woman and someone in her life: the society or environment in which she lives may also have a part to play in the onset of vaginismus. Vaginismus can, therefore, be related to wider social issues.

Situating Vaginismus in Society

While it is outside the scope of this book to discuss fully the role of women in society and how we are portrayed, these issues cannot be separated or ignored when we look at vaginismus:

> I don't think it's possible to divorce society or culture from the body image a woman has of herself. If a woman in this society has no power over her body or her life, then all she can do is say "No" with her body.
> —Anne Dickson, sexuality/assertiveness trainer and author

Much of women's experience, history and pain has gone unnoticed in the world. Indeed, this is exactly how it felt to me before I received help, when nobody seemed able to see or hear my pain about vaginismus. In the same way, women's place in society and its effects may go unnoticed in some therapeutic approaches to vaginismus.

Vaginismus and Hysteria

In 1861 Dr. Sims described vaginismus to the Obstetrical Society in London, and just three years later in Vienna Dr. Gustav Braun amputated the clitoris of a vaginismic patient. But there was worse to come: between 1859 and 1866 in London, another member of the Obstetrical Society, Dr. Isaac Baker Brown, removed the clitorides and labia of numerous women in a grotesque effort to manage their minds by regulating their bodies.[30] Baker Brown viewed this as his cure for "female insanity." Like Braun, he believed women's uncontrolled sexuality to be the major, almost defining, symptom of insanity in his Victorian clientele. In 1867 Baker Brown was expelled from the Obstetrical Society, not because of his barbaric methods but because his patients complained of trickery and coercion.[31]

In the 1800s "hysteria" became the quintessential female malady, the name deriving from the Greek *hysteron* (womb), and it thereafter assumed a central role in psychiatric dialogue.[32] In her book *The Female Malady* Elaine Showalter explains how psychiatrists and gynecologists alike interpreted madness in women, but stresses that insanity is a consequence of—rather than a deviation from—the traditional female role.[33] Then, as now, men dominated psychiatry, and doctors judged their female patients hysterical when they attempted to compete with men instead of serving them.

Apart from Jeffrey M. Masson's *A Dark Science*, I have been unable to find any descriptions of the "therapeutic" practices some doctors used to bring vaginismic women to their senses. However, I have absolutely no doubt that women suffering from this condition were seen by gynecologists or psychiatrists, diagnosed as hysterics and treated accordingly. (At the time of his expulsion from the Obstetrical Society, Baker Brown insisted that other eminent gynecologists were performing similar operations to cure hysteria.) No doubt many vaginismic women underwent horrific surgery by Dr. Baker Brown, as J.P. did at the hands of his Viennese counterpart, Dr. Braun. *The Female Malady* painfully demonstrates how cultural ideas and stereotypes about "proper" feminine behavior have shaped the definition and treatment of female insanity. This has resulted in women's emotional disorders being given specifically sexual connotations.[34]

Freud's Patriarchal View

During my research I became resentful toward and upset by prefeminist analytical writings which do not acknowledge a girl's difficulty in entering the social world without the encouragement and ability to achieve autonomy enjoyed by her brother. The mother's social conditioning and the way it influences her daughter's psychological makeup are also rarely mentioned. Since this relationship is central to our development it would seem crucial not to ignore the fact that the mother's conditioning was influenced by her parents, who themselves were products of a society which also put many constraints on women.

> Although social factors are entirely entwined in a woman's development, it is the particulars of an individual that are going to be affected. However, that child is growing up in a culture within a family, and that culture, that family and that mother's feelings and behaviors are determined by the structure of our society.
>
> —Susie Orbach

The feminist approach to therapy does not simply reject Freudian★ concepts. Rather, it embodies most traditional theories but also views woman's position in society and its effects on her emotional makeup. Feminist therapists believe social factors should not be ignored, mainly because viewing a girl's psychosexual development through the eyes of a patriarchy may risk missing the total picture of her development and predisposition to vaginismus. This might, for example, take the form of indiscriminately viewing the father, as Freud did, as the central figure in every girl's psychological development.

★ Freud's theories and concepts remain the cornerstone of all psychotherapies, and his contribution to the understanding of men and women's psychology has been invaluable. However, Freud was very much a product of his time, and it is precisely his Victorian background which is believed to have influenced and colored his view of women.

As we will see in discussing Jenny's treatment in Chapter Five, feminist therapy takes the lead from the client and finds itself ultimately concentrating on the complex issues surrounding the mother-daughter relationship. A feminist approach tends to refrain from describing a sufferer as "immature" or "childish." This approach also does not believe, as Freud did, that instinctual drives toward sex and aggression shape our psychology. It is believed that the drive is far more for intimacy and love, for relationships with other human beings. Feminist understanding of a woman's psychology centers around the knowledge that we are expected to be emotionally dependent on others, yet paradoxically find ourselves deferring to and nurturing them. One of the inevitable results of this is the ambivalent and unsatisfying feelings that may be transmitted from mother to daughter. Consequently, inside both mother and infant remains the little girl whose needs for nurturing and acceptance are never fully met.

Vaginismus as the Body's Protest

My need to understand and explain vaginismus led me to an interest in the origins of women's other problems. One in particular seems similar to vaginismus: anorexia nervosa. We might even call vaginismus genital anorexia. In her book *Hunger Strike*, Susie Orbach also sees a link between these two. She writes that although the makeup of a particular woman's psychology predisposes her to develop anorexia, she might not have developed it had she lived in a different period. Her psychology may have more in common with the preorgasmic or "frigid" woman described two or three decades ago. Such women were unable to experience sexual pleasure, expressing this in a withdrawn attitude, involuntary closedness and, in the extreme, the inability to open up and let go both psychologically and physically. The symptom of vaginismus may be the solution that our psychological makeup has sought as a defense.[35]

Hunger Strike further explains why women use their bodies to express a protest:

> We see that living within prescribed boundaries is the reason why our bodies become the vehicle for a whole range of expressions that have no other medium . . . we are forced to speak with our bodies. Whenever woman's spirit has been threatened, we have taken control of our bodies as an avenue of self-expression. If her body is the site of her protest, then equally her body is the ground on which the attempt for control is fought.[36]

The sexuality of the contemporary woman is allegedly not so constrained as in Freud's time or the 1950s, but similar social and psychological factors may be causing women to suffer a kind of spasm when eating. Perhaps this is because the desirable image of a woman's body is today based more on thinness than it ever was in Freud's era.

> Women don't have social equality. Men have a place in the world where they've been brought up to be expansive and go out and do things. Women have been consistently told to constrain themselves. To constrain the vagina is the consequence of that constraint.
>
> —Susie Orbach

> Women are still second-class citizens and it has made women contract.
>
> —Sarah

Feminist approaches to eating disorders have led the way in working therapeutically with such problems. This same approach can help the vaginismic woman look at why she is unable to allow penetration, what it means to her, and the social pressures placed on her.

In a feminist context the symptoms of anorexia nervosa and vaginismus are seen to be the body's way of protesting that a woman's needs for love, comfort, security and acceptance have never been fully met. However, it may be far more complex than this. Returning for a moment to the section of this chapter called "Good Mother, Bad Mother" (page 65), it may not simply be that the baby's needs have gone unmet so much as that a disturbance in the developing psychological processes has caused the baby to feel that love and care are unavailable to her. Her anger and frustration at not being able to feel the love may thus obliterate the genuinely loving responses that her mother may offer.

Creating a Defensive Boundary

It is not only feminists who believe that vaginismus may be connected with women's social and political status. Freud, too, was aware that social influences play a part in the construction of the feminine personality.[37] If we look at vaginismus in this wider context, as Susie Orbach looks at anorexia nervosa, it could be suggested that vaginismus illustrates the effects of a patriarchal society on us, namely our fear of being invaded by men and of losing our identity. To prevent this invasion we create a defensive boundary using our bodies, the one boundary we feel certain about. Unconsciously we see intercourse as the penetration of our boundaries, and the protection from invasion manifests physically in vaginismus.[38]

Bodily Insecurity

But how do social constraints on a woman lead to vaginismus? The impact of a patriarchal society on the mother-daughter relationship is profound and may provide the key to the development of vaginismus. If the mother is the unconscious transmitter of an "inferior" psychology of women, then this is where, as little girls, women first learned what their social role would be. This process occurred at the same time that girls were developing a psychological sense of themselves. Because of my mother's position in the world, it was hard for her to give me feelings that my body was an acceptable and safe place in which to live, develop and be expansive:

> Our mothers were rarely brought up to like sex. Thus they didn't have any way to transmit that sex is all right to the next generation. Our generation has the message that sex is OK, but it doesn't feel OK.
>
> —Susie Orbach

A mother may already be very hesitant about her daughter's exploration of her vagina. If a mother has grown up with negative ideas about the "curse," images of slimness, and a submission to sex and dominance, she must unconsciously convey to her daughter that she, too, will have to watch out in these areas. Could it be that the same social forces are at work between mothers and daughters which make particular women susceptible to vaginismus, just as others are to anorexia nervosa?

Women and the Media

Advertisements, magazines, TV and films bombard men and women with images of how women should feel, look and act, sexually and otherwise:

> Socially we are supposed to have penetrative sex at an increasingly younger age.
>
> —Dr. Patricia Gillan, psychologist

We are visually stereotyped as "perfect" and "available." Could the woman with vaginismus be unconsciously expressing her protest against such images, her desire not to compete with them, and her consequent refusal to allow any (as she sees it) dominating force inside her? So, too, if society's unconscious messages to women are always "don't do this" and "mustn't do that," could vaginismus be the only protest we feel we can make against allowing something inside us unless it is on our own terms?

Female Sexuality and Intercourse

A Dutch "emancipatory therapist" (one who seeks to work totally outside social constraints imposed on women by convention) reports on research into women's attitudes toward penetration.[39] One study reveals that approximately two thirds of happily married women wish to change their love patterns, that is, to have less intercourse, make love in ways not immediately directed to penetration, and enjoy more warmth and involvement with their partners. Some women said they never initiated sex for fear of intercourse, and we are speaking here about nonvaginismic women! Further research reveals hierarchies of preferences during love-making. Highest on the list were emotional experiences, feeling accepted and loved by the partner and an ability to love and be oneself. Much less important was penetration.* These findings imply that there is little difference between the way vaginismic and nonvaginismic women feel about penetration, in that we all need to feel known, loved and accepted before allowing anyone inside us.† In this way the gap closes between a woman who has vaginismus and one who does not.

Men's sexual likes are often stereotyped and so appear to differ from women's, with warmth, involvement and the expression of words of love generally having far more importance for us than for men. However, it may be that the intimate relationship between infant daughter and caregiver is difficult to negotiate and quite different from that between mother and son, leading us to feel unknown, unloved, un-

* My feeling is that this reported disinterest in penetration should not be interpreted literally as a dislike of intercourse. Perhaps what the research reflects more is a woman's inability to feel loved, and naturally this might make her unhappy about letting a penis inside her.
† When my body said "no" to my partner this did not necessarily mean he was the person I felt didn't know, love or accept me. Such unconscious feelings stemmed from much earlier relationships, with my mother and father.

lovable and unaccepted.* Because of this, our psychology
develops differently from men's, which may be the reason
that it seems less important for a man to need to love and
feel loved before engaging in intercourse.

Do Social Factors Influence Vaginismus?

The ideas developed by some feminist therapists clearly suggest that social forces may contribute to the occurrence of
vaginismus. Our status in an oppressed world may certainly
compound our vulnerability to vaginismus and also potentially damage the mother–daughter relationship.

The mother's social conditioning combined with her psychology may make it painfully difficult or even impossible
for her to allow her daughter the rightfulness of her needs,
her entitlement to love and security, and ownership of her
vagina.

PHYSICAL CAUSES

Excluding any deformities of the vagina such as an abnormally small vaginal opening ("introitus") or even the absence
of an opening, there may be a physical reason for the onset
of vaginismus.

For example, the condition may develop after a long period
of undiagnosed and consequently untreated painful intercourse. (The causes and treatment of dyspareunia have been
described in Chapter Two, page 13.)

Here two doctors describe how vaginismus can stem from
something physiological, such as viral warts, infections, and
so on:

* For a deeper understanding of an infant girl's developing sense of self and boundaries, I suggest reading *Understanding Women* by Susie Orbach and Luise Eichenbaum,
and also the chapter "Breeding of Body Insecurity" in Susie Orbach's *Hunger Strike*.

Untreated dyspareunia is going to end up in vaginismus quite
often. It might have been an infection of thrush which would
make intercourse painful, and from then on there's spasm.
Vaginismus is also very common after the birth of a baby.
                                        —Dr. Robina Thexton

Since gynecologists are not trained in sexuality, there are a
lot of misdiagnoses in the area of vaginismus. In order to
obtain the right treatment a woman may have to "hop" between a gynecologist who has an infectious diseases background and a therapist. This is because even when the
vaginismus is due to physical causes it may still have a psychological component, and vice versa.
  —Dr. Vicki Hufnagel, M. D. medical director,
    Institute for Reproductive Health and Center for
    Female Reconstructive Surgery, Los Angeles, California,
    and author of No More Hysterectomies

But how does an infection cause vaginismus? It is simply
that anticipation of pain during penetration can lead to the
condition. If, however, the pain continues even after the local
infection has been treated and there is still no physical explanation for it, it is possible the vaginismus is being sustained
by psychological conflicts and requires psychotherapeutic
treatment.

Vaginismus is, therefore, generally developmental; its
causes are predominantly psychological, rarely physical.

Chapter 4

SEEKING
HELP

Because vaginismus can range from mild to severe, the degree of help necessary to resolve it will also vary.

> Depending upon the causes, some women can resolve vaginismus themselves. They might, for instance, resolve it with a very understanding partner.
> —Barbara Lamb, nurse-psychosexual counselor

CAN VAGINISMUS BE RESOLVED WITHOUT PROFESSIONAL HELP?

Carol was able to resolve her vaginismus herself. She explains that her mother terrified her about becoming pregnant before she was married, and Carol believes she developed vaginismus as a consequence. After a series of unconsummated relationships she suddenly stopped worrying about becoming pregnant and, as a result, found herself able to allow complete intercourse with her next lover. She concludes:

> In my case all I did in the end was to stop worrying . . . it was a shame it took me so long.

One leading women's magazine in the United Kingdom produced a leaflet on vaginismus, beautifully written by a sensitive gynecologist.[1] The leaflet guides a woman step by step through a self-discovery exercise to help her gain confidence, in stages, that her vagina is neither small nor abnormal, and to help her familiarize herself with this often mysterious part of her body. Unlike the penis, the vagina is partly concealed, so even many women who do not have vaginismus may harbor irrational fears about its nature. Such fears do not mean these women are seriously disturbed; it is only when fear becomes so exaggerated that it prevents penetration that it needs to be explored. It is important, though, to be aware that for some of us, self-examination may not provide the final answer in resolving vaginismus. Jean describes her difficulties even after she was able to explore her vagina:

> The specialist taught me how to explore inside myself . . . I could do it when she was there, but not at home. I still remained terrified of a penis and a tampon, despite this, so the treatment fizzled out again . . . I felt it was my fault.

Exploration and educational techniques by themselves can be superficial and may not resolve vaginismus if the woman's fantasies have not been sufficiently understood and worked through. This demonstrates the gap between approaches which focus heavily on relaxing the vagina and those which do not. There may be little value in obeying a command to examine ourselves when the emotional wounds and defenses behind the vaginismus have not been sufficiently healed. Once the therapeutic process has given a woman understanding and acceptance of and comfort with herself, she may find that the desire to explore her vagina comes naturally. Such examination requires a degree of self-love and trust. (See in Part III of Chapter Five, "The Pelvic Examination" and "Self-Exploration and Self-Examination," page 201.)

The knowledge that fantasies and fears about intimacy, love and dependence stand in the way of a woman's ability to allow penetration, and *not* her smallness or tightness, is a far more meaningful acquisition in the long run than simply learning to relax her vagina because she has been given a specific instruction to do so.

WHEN SHOULD YOU SEEK HELP?

> My advice is to seek help as soon as possible . . . my vaginismus hung over me like a black cloud.
>
> —Sarah

Unfortunately, if left untreated vaginismus may persist indefinitely. My advice, therefore, is to seek help at the earliest opportunity. If the condition remains untreated, the subsequent stress may only increase.

All the doctors and therapists I consulted during the preparation of this book stressed the importance of seeking help early. One said that without intervention vaginismus often gets worse. Most expressed concern that the sufferer should feel she is not alone in her struggle. However, as explained earlier, seeking help is not always an easy step to take. It is painful to reveal to someone else that you have vaginismus, but it can feel devastating to reveal it to someone who lacks an understanding of the deep distress the condition creates. Psychotherapist Jill Curtis told me how difficult it can be for a woman to come forward after so many years of pain. Clearly, she understands our fear of seeking help:

> A lot of women have become embedded into the condition and might feel there's no hope anyway. If they do reach out, we are asking a lot of them. She is going to be afraid of being hurt, of being penetrated, and it's asking a lot of women to trust, and that's what psychotherapy is about.

Once a woman has made the decision to seek help, she has taken the first step toward resolution. However, this alone will not be enough to produce the desired change. She must be willing to become an active participant in the healing process. In attempts to relieve myself of the responsibility to overcome vaginismus, I would fantasize about being seduced and penetrated by a complete stranger, indicating an illusory belief that someone else out there could "do it to me" and "solve it for me." In this way I became the passive recipient of a "cure" rather than actively contributing to a solution. It was when I recognized how I closed up, went into spasm and could not take charge that I became more committed to my therapy and began to take responsibility for its success.

OBSTACLES THAT CREATE OPPORTUNITIES

We have all read stories in the press about professional misconduct by a doctor with a patient. Happily, cases such as these are rare. What is sadly more common is the cold, rushed and indifferent attitude of many general practitioners and hospital doctors. This may be the result of overwork, but the fact remains that I, and many other sufferers, have experienced insufficient care and attention along the way. During the writing of this book I met and corresponded with many sufferers. Painfully I listened to them recount their stories of misery, hopelessness, perseverance and courage. Often the themes echoed my own.

This is not to imply that skilled, sensitive and effective help is unavailable to women with vaginismus. The practitioners who have shared their expertise so freely in this book certainly do not represent the practices, attitudes and responses of uncaring professionals. Nevertheless, I include the painful experiences of some women because assuming that we will encounter no problems when seeking help may lull us into thinking that sensitive aid is always just around the corner. In reality it may be an uphill struggle.

> I went to so many doctors I can't remember all of them. We kept saying "Help! We can't make love," . . . but there was no treatment offered.
>
> —Jan

After a disastrous and tearful honeymoon I went to my GP. He was old, deaf and out of touch, and everyone in the waiting room could hear while I sobbed out my story. He gave me tranquilizers, but they didn't work.

—Jean

Sadly, the path toward help for my condition led to many dead ends, with my hopes being dashed and my suspicions that vaginismus was too great a problem for anyone to deal with being confirmed. I hope my experience will enable you—unlike me—to make a speedy, assertive and well-informed choice.

Because I didn't know I had vaginismus, I didn't know how or from whom I should seek help, so in 1977 I contacted a women's health clinic. My first appointment was with a gynecologist, as at the time the clinic did not employ anyone trained in psychosexual medicine. I was nervous—terrified. Although the doctor seemed to know what vaginismus was, he did not know how to explore with me the underlying causes, or how to treat it. Instead, his advice was simply to go away, relax and not worry too much, "because I don't know if you know this, but even animals find intercourse painful." Not surprisingly, I left feeling hopeless and totally confused. As I made my way to the subway station I felt overwhelmed with despair and pain. I'd gone to a doctor—a woman's doctor—for help with vaginismus. Instead, I had not been seen, heard or understood at all, but rather had been given a bizarre suggestion about the way in which animals have sex. As the train approached the platform I very nearly threw myself underneath it.

The first doctor I saw sent me away with a huge medical textbook on vaginismus with no offer of treatment. Because I was on antidepressants the book was quite beyond my comprehension. All I can remember thinking is "God, somebody else must have this," . . . knowing that I wasn't alone.

—Jan

The following month I returned to the clinic and saw a different gynecologist. Although he was kind and sympathetic and wanted to comfort me as I cried, he did not seem to grasp what vaginismus was at all, and reassuringly said, "Oh, it's very common to fear sex for the first time, in fact my own wife did. Just relax and leave it all up to your husband and it'll be fine." He then promptly wrote me six months' prescription for the Pill. On my way home I wept and thought I was probably the only woman swallowing contraceptive pills who couldn't have sex.

Several years elapsed and I returned to the clinic again, this time seeing a more enlightened gynecologist. Her planned "behavioral" treatment was to insert glass phalluses ("dilators") of graduating size into my vagina until I could tolerate one the size of an erect penis. However, the severity of my vaginismus meant that I was phobic about anything entering me and could not tolerate a pelvic examination even allowing the tip of her finger.

Eventually, the doctor decided she could only examine me while I was anesthetized. The entire experience of being intravenously sedated and then later being unable to remember the insertion of the speculum (the metal or plastic instrument used to dilate the vagina for examination) felt so brutal that I was not able to return to the clinic, or to seek help from anyone else, until more than two years later.

Unrelenting, the vaginismus continued, and in a final desperate attempt I contacted the clinic again in late 1981. This time I was very lucky. A doctor trained in family planning and psychosexual problems, who was also an analytical psychotherapist, was doing part-time psychosexual sessions at the clinic. During our first meeting we established that his approach would be to explore my feelings and fears, not my vagina. This was a turning point—not just because at last I had discovered a method which felt more right than anything I had previously encountered, but also because this doctor's attitude was so totally different. When I wept he did not just reassure me to stop me from crying. Instead he acknowledged the pain and distress I was feeling and expressed his commitment to helping me. For the first time I felt emotionally "held" and understood.

THE ABILITY TO HEAR A WOMAN'S PAIN

This doctor was hearing my pain. He did not say to me "There, there, it'll be all right," or "It's not that awful; after all, penetration isn't everything." That would have been tantamount to telling me that my problem wasn't that serious. Rather, my pain was validated because the doctor didn't rush in with the usual comforting clichés. He simply heard how terrible vaginismus made me feel in a way that no other doctor had heard it before.

We made an appointment to meet the following week, and I sensed for the first time in my life that a positive step toward resolving my vaginismus had been taken that day. Jan echoes my relief at finding the right therapist:

> When I finally saw the clinical psychologist it was incredible. We worked through the past. . . . I actually became the child.

Sadly, others have not been as fortunate. Many women simply give up searching for help after suffering repeated inappropriate responses to their vaginismus, as these comments illustrate:

> I went to family planning next. They tried to examine me but were nonplussed at my terror and just said it'd all sort itself out.

> I sobbed out my story to a marriage counselor. She was young and suburban, and hadn't a clue.

> I paid privately out of my small salary to see a psychiatrist. It was no help. He went in for long silences, which I found threatening.

The doctor at the gynecological clinic I was sent to was under pressure and rushed. He felt I was being willfully awkward and shouted at me when he couldn't examine me.

The nurses were silently accusing . . . thinking me very odd. One doctor, when she found she couldn't give me an internal, slapped my legs and told me to come back when I'd grown up.

The last specialist I saw, three years ago, just thoroughly humiliated me. I felt so belittled I vowed never to go anywhere again.

Echoing these experiences, one psychosexual therapist reports similar experiences of patients. She told me that one woman first consulted her GP because of a vaginal discharge, but when the vaginismus prevented him from examining her he became so angry he sent her away. The woman then met with a very impatient family planning doctor who was also unable to examine her. Finally, as a last resort, she consulted a specialist who gave her a general anesthetic and took a smear. The anesthetic only reinforced the woman's idea that no one could go near her vagina without her being knocked out. Though she is now receiving appropriate counseling therapy, the therapist says this last procedure set the patient back even further.

Unconscious processes at work in both sufferer and doctor can contribute to our misery. For example, why in many cases is the woman not given information about the results of the procedures? If drugs are used to reach a woman's unconscious and the findings remain unexplained and undiscussed, she may assume that there must be something deeply disturbing about what the doctor has discovered, compounding her despair even further. Jean tells of the time she was intravenously sedated and the fear she felt afterward about what she had involuntarily revealed:

The psychiatrist took me into his clinic and gave me Demerol★ . . . wonderful! . . . I could have done anything! I talked totally uninhibitedly . . . heaven knows what I said or what they made of it. I was afraid to ask, and they didn't tell me, probably assuming I was afraid to know.

Jan describes how she felt hopeless partly because a gynecologist had given her the impression that there was no hope:

He performed an internal under anesthesia and confirmed vaginismus . . . but again he didn't refer me for help. That was the end of the discussion, so this compounded the feeling in me that I had vaginismus for life.

As we look back, it would have been far better if all of us had known in the first place how to make contact with the people we worked with eventually. It might have saved us years of wasted time and unnecessary pain and anguish. Still, I wonder whether the difficult road I took helped me in the end to see what treatments were wrong for me and which were right. Maybe even the act of seeking help can be seen as part of the process rather than as a means to an end in itself.

THE IMPORTANCE OF MAKING AN INFORMED CHOICE

I wish I'd been given a choice . . . I would've chosen to see a sex therapist. I saw a program on TV and liked the understanding and talking through rather than (as in my case) just being stretched under anesthetic and given dilators to take home and use.

—Sarah

As the causes are many and the degrees of vaginismus various, there can be no single way to help a sufferer. Each

★ A trademarked analgesic (a painkiller known as Pethidine in the U.K.) administered by injection into a muscle that can make a patient feel "high."

of us responds to a special combination of therapeutic treatments. At best, several techniques for treating vaginismus can be used, and an imaginative doctor or therapist—of the sort I hope many of you will be fortunate to work with—will often amalgamate what he or she thinks will work most successfully with the individual. Because there is no one definitive course of treatment, the methods used vary from hospital to hospital, clinic to clinic, doctor to doctor—not only in technique, but also in quality. In view of the difficult and lengthy course I had to steer to find appropriate help, I cannot overemphasize the importance of knowing what treatments are available and where. I hope this helps broaden the choices for you.

The most appropriate forms of treatment for vaginismus tend to involve psychotherapeutic technique (known as the "talking treatment"). This method employs verbal communication rather than drugs or surgery. The process of talking can unlock the hidden part of the vaginismic woman's psyche which unconsciously controls the muscles in her vagina. Although psychotherapy was originally developed to treat individuals, it has now also been successfully adapted to treat couples.

> Psychotherapy *can* have a part to play in the resolution of vaginismus, but I think it can't be seen as a cure-all. I'm always very worried about psychotherapy being seen like that. I am certain, though, it could help many women reach their potential [and] can then lead to a resolution.
>
> —Jill Curtis, psychotherapist

THE IMPORTANCE OF A PROFESSIONAL ORGANIZATION

> My worry is for people who go to unqualified therapists, because at the moment there is nothing to stop anyone from advertising in magazines.
>
> —Jill Curtis

Just as you would expect a doctor or a lawyer to be qualified, expect the same of a therapist. Anyone can advertise himself or herself as a psychotherapist, sex therapist or hypnotherapist in magazines and newspapers without specified training, subjection to a code of practice or inclusion in a central register of practitioners. One British psychotherapist shared her concern with me about this situation and said that a conference has been meeting annually over the course of several years to try to achieve agreement about the description of the profession of psychotherapy; members have recently agreed to organize themselves according to their major specialties. The ultimate aim of the conference is to compile a code of ethics and a list of therapists. As this is still some years away,★ my advice is to guard your own interests until such guidelines become legal.

The safest routes to obtaining help are generally through personal recommendation, your general practitioner, or a recognized organization (see Appendix). The fact that a therapist is a member of an organization is some guarantee of competence and can also minimize the risk of exploitation. A therapist can take advantage of a woman's sexual and emotional vulnerability if he has not been sufficiently trained or if his motives are not wholly honorable. In the psychotherapeutic setting a woman may share her intimate fears and fantasies; sometimes erotic feelings will be aroused. It is important that a therapist have integrity and belong to an organization where he will be subject to some degree of regulation by his colleagues.

How does a woman avoid the person who may lack the necessary experience and qualifications? While there is no

★ As I write this in June 1991, Dr. Michael R. Pokorny, psychoanalyst and psychotherapist and chairman of the UK Standing Conference for Psychotherapy, confirms the following. Proposals for accrediting training courses are under discussion with a commitment to agree on accreditation in January 1992, so that a Register of Psychotherapists can be constructed. This should appear during the second half of 1993 and will be available to the public.

foolproof method, there are some measures a woman can take, as explained by consulting clinical psychologist Dr. Paul Brown:

> Any woman approaching a person who has got some expertise in a basic professional skill (such as doctor, social worker or psychologist) and who has also got some special interest in sexual difficulties can regard that such a person will be competent. Anyone who is advertising his services about *curing* clinical problems should be avoided like the plague.

To ensure that the right course of therapy is undertaken, a woman should generally seek an initial assessment before committing to any particular method. This consultation offers the woman the opportunity to meet with a therapist who may not be personally treating her but who will talk over with her whether in his opinion therapy will help. The aim is to try and work out what is best for the patient. Contacting an institute, society or association of recognized practitioners ensures that an initial assessment will be offered as a matter of policy; this might not be the case if a woman responded to a therapist's advertisement.

As we should take care not to pigeonhole the sufferer, so we should not hold preconceived ideas about the best person with whom to seek treatment. It does not necessarily follow that because the origins of vaginismus might lie in early development, a woman needs to seek the help of a psychoanalyst:

> The most important thing always, in anything to do with one's emotions, is to go to someone you feel will listen in a knowledgeable, caring way so that a woman can say what she wants to in her own time.
>
> —Lorna Guthrie, Jungian analyst

As the psychiatrist Dr. M. Scott Peck points out in *The Road Less Traveled*:

> A therapist's ability bears very little relationship to any cre-
> dentials he or she might have. Love and courage and wisdom
> cannot be certified by academic degrees.[2]

As well as ensuring that a person is sufficiently qualified, it
is equally important for the woman to trust her feelings and
use her intuition when choosing a therapist. I knew from the
first consultation that my analyst felt right for me. While
qualifications and standards are of course important, in such
a potentially crucial and intimate relationship a woman's
choice should be based more on her own intuitive feeling
about the person than on impressive credentials or a presti-
gious office.

> It's very important that in seeking help a woman finds the
> person she trusts. She should choose her therapist as much as
> the therapist says he can help her.
>
> —Dr. Paul Brown

The earlier help is sought, the better. Likewise, the more
informed the choice, the easier it will be to actively participate
in the healing process.

WHO TREATS VAGINISMUS?

Nowhere is the relationship between a woman and her doctor
more important than in the treatment of vaginismus. It requires a degree of trust and openness to allow someone into
one's innermost thoughts and feelings. Many vaginismic
women consciously and unconsciously attempt to keep people out. These defenses not only protect us, but also keep out
the people we love, want and need from the hidden part of
ourselves which we feel is destructive, devouring and bad.
The doctor or therapist may come up against the same defenses. Although professional qualifications are important, in
the end a person's sensitivity, experience and awareness will
do more to shape the quality of the relationship between
sufferer and helper. Much evidence exists to support the view

that it is not the type of therapy that is crucial to the success or failure of a treatment . . . it is the therapist.

A range of professionals from varied disciplines treat vaginismus. Since vaginismus may be a symptom of other, deeper conflicts, it is important that the people sufferers work with can assess the treatment possibilities. If, for example, vaginismus is not helped by self-exploration or reassurance, the skills of a therapist are essential, since examination of the less conscious factors behind the condition is a highly technical and professional business.[3] Anyone who treats vaginismus, therefore, needs to have psychotherapy skills as well as extensive knowledge of human emotions and behavior. In fact, sexual therapy should always be taught in addition to, not in place of, other basic psychotherapeutic skills, since mind and body are interrelated. A therapist should ideally always put the woman's needs first and adjust his or her method to suit each individual. It's quite possible, for example, that a psychoanalyst might refer a patient to a behavioral therapist (or vice versa) if he or she thought it would be a more appropriate way of treating her vaginismus.

The various professionals who may treat vaginismus are listed below. They will not necessarily have special expertise in treating vaginismus, so it's best to check first whether this is an area in which a particular person is happy to work. I also list the additional qualifications a professional should have if he or she is to treat vaginismus.

- Analytical psychologist or analytical psychotherapist—a medically or nonmedically qualified person with experience in psychology, social work or related fields with training in analytical psychotherapy, who has undergone his or her own psychoanalysis.

- Behavioral therapist—a psychologist with training in psychosexual problems.

- General practitioner or gynecologist—a physician who also has special interest or training in psychosexual problems.

- Homeopath—a person accredited in homeopathy who may have medical, nonmedical or nursing training, and is a member of a recognized organization.

- Hypnotherapist—a licensed physician or psychologist with evidence of training in clinical hypnosis from a recognized university, institute or professional society. In addition, a hypnotherapist should belong to one of the recognized associations, for instance New York's Institute for Research in Hypnosis and Psychotherapy or in the U.K., the Society of Medical & Dental Hypnosis or the British Society of Experimental and Clinical Hypnosis (See Appendix for details).

- Psychiatrist—a physician who also has special interest or training in psychosexual problems.

- Psychoanalyst—a psychiatrist with psychoanalytic training, who has undergone his or her own psychoanalysis.

- Psychotherapist—a physician, psychiatric social worker, psychologist, or an expert in related fields with training in psychotherapy.

- Sex therapist—a psychologist, marriage guidance counselor, psychotherapist, family planning doctor, family planning nurse, or psychiatric social worker with training in sexual therapy.

For further reading and guidance on choosing a therapist, see *A Complete Guide to Therapy: From Psychoanalysis to Behavior Modification* by Joel Kovel, and Chapters 10 and 11 of *In Our Own Hands* by Sheila Ernst and Lucy Goodison. (See Suggested Reading, page 348.)

Chapter 5

The Treatments and How They Work

Sadly, a bit of a stigma still attaches to any psychological problem that requires therapy, and vaginismus is no exception. The misconception that you must be middle-class, rich, well-educated or neurotic to benefit from therapy may deter many from seeking the necessary help. As consumers of health services we may also find it a daunting task to select the most appropriate therapy. By describing each method as simply as possible I hope to demystify the process, dispel any unfounded myths and fears and enable you to make a choice.

No One Road to Resolution

Many of the treatments I outline may seem to blur into one another. "Sex therapy" is a generic term used to describe any method that seeks to help a woman with a sexual problem, and the Masters & Johnson approach, behavioral therapy, psychotherapy and general counseling may all be applied when treating vaginismus. There are, however, three distinct schools of psychotherapy:

- *Psychodynamic/psychoanalytic* therapy—an approach in which a woman's psychological processes and forces are studied. This therapy is generally based on the theories and techniques of Freud.

- *Behavioral/sex therapy*—an approach in which a woman's conditioning and learned behavior are studied.

- *Humanistic/growth* therapy—a method (sometimes using group work) which involves working on the body as well as the mind, with the emphasis on the spiritual side. Such therapies include Gestalt, psychodramatic, encounter and transpersonal approaches.

Even within these three schools of therapy there may often be a mixture of one, two or sometimes all three approaches. However, for the majority of sufferers from vaginismus, psychodynamic and behavioral methods are most commonly employed.

Apart from psychoanalysis with its rigid rules and guidelines, no clearly defined boundaries separate one method from another. The most successful is ideally woman-oriented, tailor-made. Perhaps the art of achieving a successful outcome is the ability to match the woman with the right therapy and therapist. As hypnotherapist Anne Mathieson says:

Many roads lead to Rome, and we have to find the right treatment for every woman.

In fact, practitioners agree on the importance of stating that vaginismus cannot be treated in any one specific way.

What we need to get away from indicating to any woman is that there's a pattern she can go through. Every single woman will have got to this [vaginismus] in a very different way, so it can't be treated the same way, either.
—Jill Curtis, psychotherapist

Some vaginismic women are rather fragile from a psychological point of view. That is, the vaginismus is a sign of other kinds of problems with fear that the woman may have. We have treated vaginismic women who have a history of other kinds of phobias and fears, or a history that includes sexual abuse, and so the treatment often needs to be broadened to cover these issues as well.

> —Dr. Marian E. Dunn,
> Director of the Center for Human Sexuality, State University of New York Health Science Center, Brooklyn

Swedish psychotherapist Marianne Granö explains that she assesses each sufferer differently and adapts her method accordingly:

> There is no set way I work with a woman. With some, I decide very early on to try and encourage them to examine themselves, but with others I would not be working in the same way.

FINANCIAL CONSIDERATIONS

Medical services in the United States are becoming increasingly expensive, and it may seem daunting to embark on an open-ended treatment. You may also feel it is terribly unjust that not only are you suffering emotionally but you will also have to suffer financially.

Individual therapists and counselors may have negotiable fees, and some treatment centers offer a sliding payment scale. If you have limited money or lack medical insurance, you may be able to seek assistance at a government- or hospital-supported psychiatric or mental health clinic where the fees will be set according to your means. This requires some research on your part. Alternatively, you could ask a psychiatrist to refer you to a less expensive, nonmedical therapist, if appropriate. A good psychiatrist should be happy to tell you about competent practitioners. Word-of-mouth recommendation is also a reliable way to get started; perhaps a friend has had a positive experience with a gynecologist or general practitioner. However, bear in mind that a practitioner suited to a friend may not be the right person for you.

What Should Determine the Treatment?

The choice of a method depends on many factors, but probably the way a woman perceives her vaginismus should be the ultimate determinant in her decision. If, for example, she sees it as a purely learned or purely sexual problem, behavioral treatments, which focus heavily on the symptom, will be much more appropriate. However, if, like me, she sees vaginismus as not being separate from her but part of a much deeper personality conflict, psychodynamic or psychoanalytic therapies, which aim to give the client insight into her psychology, will probably be more suited.

This aspect is better explained by Dr. Paul Brown, a practicing psychologist with expertise in assessing patients:

> It's important diagnostically to distinguish between women who are fairly integrated about their sexuality and whose vaginismus often relates to very clear trauma they might have had experience of. There will be a lot of uncertainty or distress about the vagina and they just feel they can't relax enough to allow penetration to happen. This group is relatively simple to treat, and typically women respond to behavioral programs quite quickly. There is another group where the unconscious forces are much more in evidence, with deep fears about what is going on inside them. This requires much more aware and sympathetic psychotherapy. Distinguishing between these two groups gives some clues as to what treatment method one is going to use, and the approach should be defined fairly early on.

Considering the diversity of women's personalities and experience, the question of what therapy is most effective is far better left open, since this encourages seeing people as individuals. We should avoid trying to fit a woman to a treatment simply because it has been voted the most successful in treating vaginismus. It is far more desirable to try and fit the therapy to the woman.

Before taking a look at what happens in the therapist's office, I want to mention that the order in which the treatments are described is based on their availability and the commonness with which they are employed in treating vaginismus; their order does not reflect in any way my preference or the methods' rates of success. For example, my own form of treatment appears toward the end of this section simply because vaginismus is not very often treated by a psychoanalyst. Similarly, the treatments described, though based mainly on the experiences of women in heterosexual relationships, pertain equally to women in lesbian relationships.

While I describe the many ways in which vaginismus can be treated by a professional, this does not necessarily imply that the expertise is exclusively held by specialists. I see the treatment as a process of sharing and learning, rather than one in which the woman is a patient with little power and no sense of her own expertise. In reality, it isn't the "expert" or the treatment that counts as much as the woman's own contribution to the therapeutic partnership.

HOW TO READ THE TREATMENTS SECTION

Apart from "Linda's Treatment," which is based on my own experience of analytical psychotherapy, the names of all the sufferers in this section have been changed, and some of the case histories are composites formed from the experiences of several different women. Each example is, nonetheless, a realistic portrayal of what happens in the therapist's office. Doctors and therapists are also quoted throughout this section, but their statements do not relate directly to the patients in any of my examples.★

★ However, I have not referred to the gynecologist in "The Pelvic Examination" as "she" because the doctor who treated me was a man. Although some women prefer to see female gynecologists, their choice can often be limited; at the moment more than 90 percent of obstetric and gynecologic specialists in the U.S. and in the U.K. are men. It is hoped that an increasing number of women will choose this sensitive specialty.

Although I describe each particular treatment, my descriptions naturally cannot represent the exact way in which each will be practiced. No two women are alike, and no two therapists practice in the same way; each person brings his or her own instincts, style and creativity to his or her method. This means, for example, that you might find a psychosexual doctor practicing much more psychodynamically, or a behavioral therapist who uses some analytic technique, or a sex therapist who rarely uses direct counseling (i.e. actually giving advice) and relies almost solely on psychotherapy.

I hope these examples convey some of the flavor of the therapeutic process. However, whatever method is used to illustrate a case study, it can never truly convey the unique nature of the relationship between one human being and another who has come to him or her to be healed. A therapist may provide a kind of psychological hand-holding; may become Mother, giving us permission to enjoy sex; may play the role of the supportive teacher; or may reassure a frightened woman that the alarming fantasies and fears that live inside her will destroy neither therapist nor patient. For many of us, the therapeutic encounter may be the first time in our lives that we have someone on our side with whom we can explore painful emotions.

Equally, my examples can never convey the pain, frustration and sheer hard work that often come with the effort to resolve vaginismus. Sometimes the lack of progress or the emergence of painful feelings may become so unbearable that a woman may wish to discontinue treatment. Whatever treatment is finally undertaken, it may represent a rough road for both the woman and the therapist, and it may also be a long road: a condition a woman has suffered from for a large part of her life may well take a number of years to resolve. Each method described here, while it takes up only a few pages, will have taken place over an extended period ranging from about three months to perhaps more than seven years.

ONE-TO-ONE THERAPY

This generally involves the woman's working alone with her therapist, although her partner is sometimes required to attend some, if not all, of the sessions.

BEHAVIOR THERAPY

Behavior therapy sees vaginismus not necessarily as the result of emotional conflicts, but as a learned or conditioned reflex which has been acquired as a way of coping with a certain stressful situation. In other words, vaginismus can be resolved through unlearning and unconditioning. Although behavioral therapists are usually not concerned with the reasons that a woman has vaginismus, some psychologists have found that they can successfully combine behavioral and psychodynamic approaches in treatment.

The following case history illustrates two behavioral techniques most commonly used by doctors and psychologists who treat vaginismus. However, it should be recognized that the techniques I describe cannot in themselves be seen as a therapy; they merely form part of a treatment program.

SANDRA'S TREATMENT

Sandra was twenty-three and engaged to be married. She was still a virgin, and because she had never been able to insert tampons she believed that her vagina was abnormally small and that a tough hymen was blocking the entrance. Consequently, she was convinced that penetration would damage her. Sandra was referred to a sex therapist by her general practitioner. The sessions took place once a week in an outpatient clinic of a large hospital.

Systematic Desensitization

This is a gradual process whereby the therapist provides a graded series of experiences from the least to the most threatening. It proceeds mainly in two ways:

- The in vitro method ("in vitro" referring to a process occurring outside the body in an artificial environment): Sandra was taught how to relax during a session and was exposed to the feared situation in stages by being asked to imagine all the steps of lovemaking, including penetration. To speed this process, hypnosis may be used (see page 141). Once she could tolerate the imagery in a session, Sandra was instructed to reproduce it at home with her partner until intercourse could be attempted.

- The in vivo method ("in vivo" referring to a process occurring inside the body in a natural environment): This proceeded once Sandra felt relaxed enough to imagine erotic and sexual situations without panic. She learned how to insert a finger into her vagina and was given glass dilators to take home and insert gently into her vagina. The real purpose of the dilators was not to enlarge Sandra's vagina—since a small vaginal opening is rarely the reason for vaginismus—but to convince her that her vaginismus had been corrected and to give her confidence. The dilators became larger as the in vivo treatment progressed.

Confronting the Worst Fear ("Flooding")

The therapist explained that as part of Sandra's treatment, and with her consent, the therapist would confront Sandra with the most fearful situation she could imagine, without providing Sandra with an opportunity to escape from her feelings. This, the therapist explained, is called "flooding."

When Sandra became used to this process and could "stay with" her fears, her phobic response (vaginismus) was eventually extinguished. The theory is that once Sandra could tolerate her worst fantasy, which was her unconscious expectation of damage, she would be able to tolerate intercourse. The therapist also taught Sandra relaxation techniques to help her during this process.

Sandra's therapist used the behavioral techniques of in vitro and in vivo desensitization combined with the flooding method so that once Sandra was able to insert the largest dilator in her vagina and her phobia of penetration had been alleviated, she and her lover would be encouraged to attempt intercourse. These techniques are particularly useful in treating vaginismus, where the specific fear or phobia of penetration can impede and complicate treatment. Accordingly, some therapists may desensitize a woman before she begins sex therapy (described next).

SEX THERAPY

A form of behavioral therapy used specifically to treat sexual problems was developed in the late 1950s by Dr. William Masters, an obstetrician, and Virginia Johnson, then his researcher. Masters & Johnson believe vaginismus can be overcome quickly through intensive reeducation, as opposed to probing and lengthy individual therapy that explores the client's deeper emotional conflicts. The techniques described form the main components of most sex therapies, distinguishing them from psychotherapy and psychoanalysis. This very popular form of treatment is used by psychologists as well as sex therapy counselors. Although it is here described in stages, no therapy can be expected to conform to a set pattern or timetable. As Alison Clegg, sex therapy training officer with the Relate Marriage Guidance Council, explains:

We have an open contract and always move at the client's pace. Although we have a basic program we don't just process people through it. Each behavioral program is tailor-made for each client couple and takes account of their particular unique needs.

AMY AND ROB'S TREATMENT

Amy, twenty-seven, and Rob, twenty-nine, had been married for three years, but because of Amy's vaginismus they had not been able to consummate their marriage. Amy imagined that her vagina was too small to accommodate Rob's penis, and this led to her terror of being penetrated and "ripped apart."

Amy felt sure she was the only woman who had this problem, but in a magazine article she came across the work of Masters & Johnson. She then asked her family doctor to refer her to the Institute for treatment.

The Couple as Patient

The doctor told the couple that Rob would have to be part of the therapy, since Masters & Johnson never see vaginismus as only the woman's problem, but rather as the couple's. Accordingly, they were treated together ("conjoint therapy").

> Masters & Johnson said some simple but revolutionary things, like "Sex tends to happen between two people," which we'd never observed before. Typically we would see only one person, not the couple, with a sexual difficulty.
> —Dr. Paul Brown, consulting clinical psychologist

Selection of Patients

About 50 percent of patients are referred by health-care professionals, and 50 percent are self-referred. Amy and Rob's family doctor explained to them that because of Masters & Johnson's rule on assessing suitability of couples, they would not be accepted into the program unless they underwent an initial interview.

Intensive Treatment

Masters & Johnson believe that if sex is exposed to daily consideration, stimulation elevates rapidly. Amy and Rob's therapy was therefore part of an intensive two-week residential program. They were required to check into a hotel and were isolated from the demands of everyday life. This allowed for full concentration on resolving Amy's vaginismus. The intensity of treatment is considered important by many therapists, including Dr. Martin Cole:

> Ideally, I usually see women at weekly intervals. If you leave it too long then the motivation will drop.

Therapists Working in Pairs

Amy and Rob learned that Masters & Johnson prefer to have a male therapist working with a female (together, they are cotherapists). Having a therapist of the same gender for each partner ensured that Amy would have "a friend on her side" representing her in the joint sessions. "I prefer co-therapy because I think a woman therapist is immensely reassuring."

Family History

To ensure the success of Amy and Rob's treatment, careful separate assessments were made to ascertain whether Amy's vaginismus was primarily learned or psychological, and whether Rob had any problems with potency. If deeper roots had been suspected, counseling would have been suggested to uncover any conflicts which could have hindered the progress of the behavioral therapy.

If the vaginismus is a deeper problem, then one uses whatever counseling or psychotherapeutic strategy one feels is appropriate to get to the root of the problem.

—Dr. Paul Brown

Surrogate Partners

Masters & Johnson introduced the use of surrogates into their program in 1959. A surrogate is a lover provided by the cotherapists for people without a partner. Some women may feel quite shocked, and others quite excited, at the prospect of making love with a stranger. Perhaps surrogates have a place in treating vaginismus, but I have many reservations about them. In the past, media sensationalism and legal difficulties have often prohibited the use of surrogates. Now, however, in view of the grave concerns about AIDS, Masters & Johnson no longer provide a surrogate program. Dr. Masters explains:

> Although we certainly include an established partner in the treatment of any woman with vaginismus, it is possible to treat the distress on an individual basis with a high degree of success.

Reeducation

The existence of Amy's vaginismus was demonstrated to her and Rob, first by showing them diagrams of the involuntary reflex action (a revelation to them both) and then by a doctor's attempting to perform a vaginal examination by introducing one finger into Amy's vagina in Rob's presence.

> I make sure the woman knows her anatomy by teaching her about it, by getting her to read books. I help her understand the pelvic anatomy so that she knows the musculature.

—Dr. Paul Brown

Psychoeducation is critical. I simply explain the normality of the experience of intercourse, explaining that the muscles are not there to close her vagina, that they're there to open it. We also use video films showing women inserting dilators so she can actually see how the vagina opens up.

—Dr. Martin Cole

Kegel Exercises, Relaxation and Fantasy

Vaginal exercises known as Kegel exercises (after Dr. Arnold Kegel, the California gynecologist who devised them) are designed to help women restore muscle tone after childbirth, since it is believed that poor muscle tone can impair sexual enjoyment. Amy was instructed to contract and release a muscle in her vagina (the pubococcygeus, or PC) as if she were trying to stop the flow of urine. This demonstrated to Amy that she indeed had control over her vagina. The exercises also increased Amy's awareness of her feelings, and with the focus on pleasant new sensations she was encouraged to enjoy sexual fantasies. The aim was to help reduce anxiety and to associate pleasure (not the conditioned fear of pain) with penetration.

> I would get her into a method of relaxing. It might simply be warm baths, or I might teach her relaxation or use hypnosis to induce relaxation.
>
> —Dr. Paul Brown

> I think it's important that the woman be able to imagine herself having intercourse and being aroused.
>
> —Dr. Martin Cole, Sex Therapist

Throughout the entire program, Amy was encouraged to report on the feelings and fantasies that emerged either during or after a particular exercise or task.

Desensitization

Using in vitro and in vivo methods of desensitization (as in Sandra's treatment), dilators of graduating size were given to Amy, and she and Rob were instructed to insert them into Amy's vagina at home. After they could be introduced suc-

cessfully without anxiety, Amy was encouraged to retain the
largest dilator inside her vagina for several hours each night
to accustom her to the feeling.

> Rather than use dilators (because it introduces a foreign object)
> I prefer her to use her fingers and would suggest she explore
> the outer entrance to the vagina. Once she begins to feel safer
> and more skillful, she can go on from one finger to two. Once
> she has done this I would begin to teach her partner the same
> skills of finger insertion. It's typical that after three-finger
> insertion a woman begins to be interested in introducing an
> erection.
>
> —Dr. Paul Brown

Many therapists, like Dr. Brown, encourage the woman
to accept her own or her partner's finger(s) rather than a
foreign object. However, there may be a good reason to
suggest a dilator. Alison Clegg explains:

> We don't like the word "dilator" because it suggests that the
> vagina is too small and has to be stretched. We call them
> "vaginal trainers." The only circumstances in which we
> would introduce them is when the woman is unable to make
> the transition from fingers to penis. If she despairs at this
> point we can reassure her and offer her the trainers as another
> resource.

Sensate Focusing

Simultaneously with the other techniques, Amy and Rob
were given homework assignments in the form of erotic tasks
to be performed in private. This is called sensate focusing,
whereby the focus of sexual activity is removed from penetration by banning intercourse, and pleasure centers around
stroking, kissing, massage and caressing, with the emphasis
on the motto "sex is fun." The anxiety which so often sur-
rounds vaginismus can ultimately eliminate enjoyment from
lovemaking, so these tasks, instead of being goal-oriented
foreplay, were designed to encourage Amy and Rob to aban-
don themselves to sensations rather than strive for penetra-

tion. Only when they felt ready to embark on intercourse were they encouraged to do so. This stage generally comes after the woman is able to insert the vaginal trainers herself.

> We call the stage before intercourse the "quiet vagina" and suggest the partner lie on his back while she gets into the female superior position. In this way she feels more in control and less anxious that he will overpower her.
>
> —Alison Clegg

Amy was encouraged to attempt penetration by kneeling astride Rob and lowering herself onto his penis, which he kept still. In this way, Amy was using Rob's penis as a trainer. It was suggested that Rob should not thrust into Amy, but allow her the opportunity to experience the sensations that the presence of his penis inside her evoked. Amy was asked in the following session how it had made her feel to have Rob inside her, and Rob was asked how it had felt for him. Once penetration occurred in this way, sexual intercourse could be attempted in any position they chose, with Amy being encouraged to make the thrusting movements herself.

> I wouldn't regard the treatment of vaginismus as being complete simply because the woman can tolerate penetration. There is a big difference between tolerating penetration and being capable and skillful at making love. Being sexually competent is not just being able to relax enough to be fertilized; these days it's about appreciating one's sexuality.
>
> —Dr. Paul Brown

PSYCHOSEXUAL MEDICINE*

This is a form of sex therapy which combines therapy and gynecology, and was pioneered in 1958 by the Family Planning Association in the United Kingdom. While this form

* U.S. practitioners interested in the methods described here should contact: The Scientific Director, Institute of Psychosexual Medicine, 11 Chandos Street, Cavendish Square, London W1M 9DE England. Tel: (071) 580 0631.

of therapy has no exact American equivalent, my research confirms that individual gynecologists, physicians and therapists in the United States are practicing along very similar lines. It therefore merits inclusion here.

TINA'S TREATMENT

Tina, who was twenty-six, had been married for two years. She had always dreaded penetration and recalled hearing at school that first-time sex was always painful. Embarrassed that she hadn't had intercourse, Tina felt unable to consult her general practitioner. Instead she made an appointment with a family planning clinic on the pretext of wanting to go on the Pill. The doctor Tina saw was a member of London's Institute of Psychosexual Medicine, and she endeavored to help Tina discover for herself the nature of the block that prevented her from engaging in and enjoying intercourse.

The Doctor's Sensitivity

The doctor's training encouraged her to be sensitive to what women like Tina transmitted. When the doctor felt something, this feeling was not acted on, but was examined and understood as an indication of some underlying conflict in Tina. This required the doctor to discover her ability to listen to things that were barely being said by Tina and to begin listening to the same kind of language in herself.

> I hold an unstructured interview. In fact, I don't speak but wait for her to, so that she talks about the things that are on her mind and I encourage her to say more. I try and notice what is going on in the interaction between me and the patient, and I try to understand it. Is she treating me like a mother, or a teacher, or asking for tips and help? Those are the kinds of clues which give me an idea as to what's going on and I

can perhaps put it back to her so that she gets a better understanding of herself.

> —Dr. Robina Thexton,
> member, Institute of Psychosexual Medicine

Another doctor explains how a woman's body can "speak" for her:

> What you get with some women who have vaginismus is the same thing in a consultation that you get within her body, and that is she has an extreme difficulty in talking.
>
> —Dr. Katharine Draper

Therapeutic Use of Vaginal Examination

Attention was focused on Tina's genital difficulty, and interpretations were offered mostly at that level. Although some counseling was offered, the doctor was primarily concerned with Tina's body and, unlike psychotherapists and psychoanalysts, was prepared to examine Tina's vagina. The examination was made not only to ascertain pelvic normality, but also to create a situation in which Tina's reactions could be observed and her fears and fantasies discussed. Typically, psychosexual treatment involves the doctor's examining and talking to a woman at the same time. This approach is called psychosomatic, because the woman's mind (psyche) and body (soma) are examined together.

> All along the line I am thinking, "Is it an appropriate moment to examine this patient, and if it isn't why isn't it?" Sensitive handling of the genital examination is a very important part. The examination itself is a very vital time when we encourage her to talk about her feelings about her body, why is it tight, what is the pain? Our method is aimed at understanding what happens during this examination when the woman reveals feelings about her body.
>
> —Dr. Robina Thexton

But it isn't just the actual examination which can give clues; as Dr. Katharine Draper points out, she also observes the way a woman prepares herself for the examination:

> It's also significant how she gets on the couch. All the time the women are showing you [these] things and I can see what she is saying about her sexuality.

Encouragement to Express Fantasies and Fears

A central aspect of Tina's treatment was the encouragement to discuss her fantasies while being vaginally examined. The doctor sought to integrate the physical examination with a thorough psychological examination of Tina's emotions and imaginings, centered on her vagina and its function. It was felt that fearful, unrealistic fantasies would cease being such strong barriers against intercourse once expressed, examined and discussed openly.[1] Tina was then better able to recognize them as unrealistic and thereby ceased to be so inhibited by them.

> I take it little by little and just go on and on, in very short steps. Once we begin to make a little progress I say, "Look, I've slipped a finger in, what about you trying?" But all the time thinking about what we are doing, not just doing it like dilators and making it bigger but trying in that way to reach her ideas. Sometimes when they are on the [table] women will produce their ideas and usually we can reach them.
> —Dr. Katharine Draper

OB/GYN NURSE-PRACTITIONERS, NURSE-MIDWIVES, AND NURSE PSYCHOSEXUAL COUNSELLORS

As with all professionals, individual nurses may develop professionally in specialized areas, and these areas could include psychosexual disorders. The subject of vaginismus is covered in the course of study of all nurse-midwives. However, whether a nurse-midwife will treat vaginismus generally will depend very much on the population served, her level of comfort with psychosexual problems and the availability of other resources in the community. Advanced nurses can elect to take training at the master's degree level in family health programs, and vaginismus is included as a general part of the curriculum covering health care of women.

The combination of gynecology and communication skills gives a nurse-practitioner or nurse-therapist particular expertise in the area of vaginismus. She will have had extensive experience in the field of women's health which helps her to understand, communicate about and examine women's bodies. In the U.K. a nurse with this special training, together with recognized training in counselling, is called a nurse psychosexual counsellor.

There are many advantages in seeing a nurse as opposed to a physician:

> Because of our health education and counseling training, our individual approach is more geared toward empowering patients to make their own health decisions and manage health programs. We diagnose in the same way as doctors, but we take it one step further in providing the woman with support to make our service truly preventative. Doctors tend to be more intervention-oriented, whereas we generally start with simple ideas and move on to more complex ones only when necessary.
>
> —Mimi Clark Secor, registered nurse-practitioner

LOUISE'S TREATMENT

Louise was twenty-four and had been married for eighteen months. She came to a family planning clinic initially asking for help with infertility. She was tearful, but eventually the nurse elicited from her that the reason that she could not get pregnant was because she and her husband were unable to have intercourse. Louise explained that she had always been terrified of examining her vagina (which she described as "small, slimy and dark") and that any attempt her husband made to penetrate ended in tears and pain because her vagina clamped tightly shut.

Talking, Listening and Examining

The nurse explained to Louise that initially she would like to see her and her husband together. Louise and her husband were then seen individually, and the nurse described the treatment to each. Part of this assessment involved the nurse's listening and trying to understand what Louise was saying.

> The women have great difficulty in explaining what is wrong with them, thinking they are the only ones with this particular problem. I'm not always able to examine during the first consultation, but when the woman is in that particular position on the [table] we can eliminate quite a lot of fears, and she begins to tell quite a few things.
>
> —Barbara Lamb, nurse-psychosexual counselor

Counseling and Sensate Focusing

Louise told the nurse she felt a great relief at being able to talk about and share her anxieties with somebody who was understanding and did not laugh at her. The nurse used her skills to suit Louise's particular problems. She combined an examination of Louise's psychological problems with sensate focusing exercises to remove the pressure to accommodate penetration (as in Amy's treatment).

> I talk a lot about a woman's feelings, what are her expectations, how long has she had vaginismus. Then maybe we will do some exploration on the first visit. I think what makes my treatment successful is possibly women find it easier to relate to a nurse than a doctor. They feel very much on the same level as me.
>
> —Barbara Lamb

I feel that nurse-midwives are excellent practitioners to counsel women with vaginismus. We hear, because we ask, about many psychosexual problems that women experience, and our clients feel more relaxed with us than with a male physician.

—Marion McCartney, certified nurse-midwife

Helping a Woman to Accept and Own Her Vagina

The nurse believed she could work successfully with Louise, since the nurse saw the vaginismus as more to do with the need for Louise to come to terms with her own body than with some deep psychological problem. In some family planning clinics, a psychiatrist may work alongside psychosexual doctors and nurse-therapists. While a psychiatrist treats the psychological aspects of vaginismus, he will not examine the patient. The nurse, however, was able to treat Louise's vaginismus on a practical level without psychiatric intervention. She offered Louise self-exploration techniques to help Louise understand her vagina better.

I make it quite simple; I look at and treat much more the physical part rather than the mental side of vaginismus. But also one needs to understand *why* a woman feels she can't consummate her relationship. I do believe a woman has got to learn to examine her own body, know what vaginismus is, know that it's a muscular spasm. Know what she is doing when penetration takes place and how to avoid this happening.

—Barbara Lamb

I reassure the woman that vaginismus is a common problem, that it is due to "fear-tension-pain" syndrome, like labor, and that it's very treatable—this is my first step. Then I demonstrate during a vaginal exam using a mirror what is happening—teaching women how to tense and relax their pelvic floor muscles helps. Other suggestions—include using a good lubricant . . . , counseling the partner about not getting

overanxious or feeling rejected and encouraging the partners to talk to each other about their needs—seem to work, too.
—Marion McCartney

Guidance and Self-Help

After several sessions the nurse was able to teach Louise how to insert one, two and three fingers painlessly into her own vagina (as in Sandra's and Amy's treatments). Dilators were not used, as the nurse found that women preferred to insert either fingers or the cervical cap. She observed that women found the cap more acceptable, as it gently and naturally expands inside the vagina as it enters.

> I don't promise success overnight and explain that we have to work through it together. The couple make it work, but as the counselor I see myself as their "referee" to guide them through it. When the woman is ready to make love I usually suggest the female superior position so that she is in control.
> —Barbara Lamb

COMBINED BEHAVIORAL AND PSYCHODYNAMIC SEX THERAPY

In the field of psychosexual medicine, information and techniques are constantly evolving and improving, through both large organizations and individual practitioners. To reflect this, in the 1970s a combination of behavioral and psychodynamic methods was introduced by Dr. Helen Singer Kaplan, M.D., Ph.D., Clinical Associate Professor of Psychiatry, Cornell University College of Medicine, New York. Her treatment (known as the New Sex Therapy) is a kind of marriage between behavioral and psychodynamic techniques. Dr. Kaplan has said:

> The treatment of choice which I use consists of a combination of gradual vaginal self-dilation with a psychodynamically oriented exploration of the patient's deeper emotional conflicts

and her resistances, which does, of course, make use of doctor-patient transference.*

Kaplan's method rejects the Freudian view that unconscious conflicts are the only cause of vaginismus, and focuses on the present rather than the past. It goes one step further than Masters & Johnson because it not only uses desensitization techniques, but also attempts to make the woman's unconscious more conscious and so reduce her phobia rapidly. This combined approach aims to deal with the psychological issues as they crop up, but not in anything like the depth of psychotherapy or psychoanalysis. It may, however, help the woman with vaginismus gain simple insights into her childhood or crucial early experiences that may have contributed to the condition.

ELLEN'S TREATMENT

Ellen, thirty-five, shared an apartment with two women friends in New York City. After a five-year marriage in which she had been unable to engage in intercourse, she and her husband had separated one year earlier. Ellen had always had a fearful expectation that penetration would cause her pain and bleeding, and was referred for treatment by a psychiatrist.

Dealing with the Immediate Cause of Vaginismus

Using behavioral methods, the doctor focused initially on the "immediate" causes of Ellen's vaginismus (cited as poor relationships, ignorance and anxiety about sexual performance). If progress had not been made, then, using psychodynamic methods, the doctor would have directed her attention to the "remote" causes (responsible for the beginnings of vaginismus and usually occurring during early development or after a trauma).

* For a discussion of transference, see "Linda's Treatment," page 154.

Such treatment may often involve the doctor's actually bypassing the exploration of the deeper origins of vaginismus. Doctors like Ellen's who practice this method tend to believe that this exploration is simply not needed to resolve the condition.

> In this country, the psychoanalytic approach is not considered effective for this disorder.
>
> —Dr. Helen Singer Kaplan

Ellen was so fearful of the internal examination that she found it difficult to get onto the examination table: it can take some women a large part of the session. Once there, she found it impossible even to open her legs. They just didn't seem to be under her control. The first step, therefore, was to help Ellen learn how to relax her thigh muscles to allow the doctor access to her vulva and then eventually for the doctor to simply place one finger at the entrance to the vagina.

The marriage between the behavioral and psychodynamic approach meant that Ellen's doctor could use physical techniques to help desensitize Ellen's conditioned response to being penetrated. Glass dilators were not used (as in Sandra's and Amy's treatments). Instead, the doctor began with her finger and then progressed to vaginal trainers. The doctor also taught Ellen Kegel exercises (as with Amy) to relax her vaginal muscles and make her aware of her self-control and bodily sensations.

For the doctor, trying to insert a finger into the vagina of a patient like Ellen may feel like trying to put a finger through the center of the palm of a hand. Ellen's doctor pressed ever so slightly, without pushing her finger in. At this stage she began to teach Ellen how to tighten and loosen her vaginal muscles, never pushing her finger in against tight muscles but instead making it clear that it was only when Ellen relaxed her muscles that her finger would move. In this way, Ellen was letting in the doctor, rather than the doctor pushing her finger in.

At each stage of the examination, Ellen's doctor helped her explore her feelings. When the doctor's finger was at the entrance to Ellen's vagina, Ellen revealed a terror of being ripped apart, of a devastation of some kind . . . almost an annihilation.★ These feelings were discussed so that Ellen was finally helped to understand them.

Ellen did not attempt intercourse with her current boyfriend until she could insert a trainer into her vagina without fear or pain. Since many women with vaginismus harbor a distorted and very negative image about their bodies, with the help of the doctor Ellen learned the facts about her genital area.

Further Exploration Only When Necessary

Ellen's treatment was primarily limited to relief of her vaginismus without exploring its origins, and as such that relief had to override any other factors. The deeper (remote) causes were dealt with only when they presented an obstacle to treatment.

When a difficulty did emerge, such as Ellen's repeatedly being unable to allow the doctor's finger to enter her vagina, Ellen's doctor began to explore, interpret and analyze her resistance. If deeper conflicts had appeared to make Ellen's vaginismus harder to overcome with this approach, the doctor might have suggested individual psychotherapy.

WHO BENEFITS MOST FROM THE BEHAVIORAL, PSYCHOSEXUAL AND SEX THERAPIES?

If a woman, although apprehensive, can tolerate a one–finger examination without trauma, she will feel reassured and will have taken the first step in the therapeutic reversal of vagi-

★ For more on the idea of annihilation, see "The Beginnings" in Chapter Three, page 62; and in Chapter Five, "The Pelvic Examination," page 201, and "Self-Examination and Self-Exploration," page 210.

nismus.[2] Likewise, if she sees vaginismus as being a purely sexual difficulty, seeks quick insights without the desire for deeper changes, is keenly motivated and can recognize the link between mind and body, she may be more suited to the directive methods. However, behavioral techniques are generally employed only when the phobia of penetration is secondary to the vaginismus.

Behavior therapy works on the assumption that psychologically rooted vaginismus can be consciously isolated and treated externally with direct instructions and exercises. While this treatment might well suit the woman who sees vaginismus purely as a sexual difficulty, the woman who cannot separate the vaginismus from her other conflicts may not respond so well. If the prospect of a vaginal examination fills a woman with dread, if she needs to feel power over and control of the doctor, or if she is phobic about being touched vaginally, the physical methods employed by these treatments should not be undertaken. Any severe anxieties which continue to prevent an examination should be taken as an indicator that the woman needs to explore the underlying conflicts to bring about resolution of vaginismus.

> If the emotional block is so deep-seated, then possibly nobody is going to get to it unless the woman receives a full psychoanalysis. I would try and refer her on after an interval. Sometimes the woman gets despairing about the lack of movement and she drops out of treatment. Maybe her need to stay in control of her body, the muscle and her life is so strong, but I always hope to have pointed that out to her before we part. If she doesn't turn up for treatment then I write her a letter about it so that we try and get it out in the open.
>
> —Dr. Robina Thexton

I share Masters and Johnson's view that it is brutal to put a woman in a situation which might severely traumatize her. If an internal examination can only be accomplished by force, clearly this approach must be discarded. The resultant trauma could make vaginismus even more difficult to treat.[3]

HYPNOTHERAPY

As with the desensitization techniques in Sandra's treatment, hypnosis alone should not be viewed as a complete therapy for vaginismus. Rather, it is generally used in addition to a physician's or therapist's other methods. Accordingly, it would not be appropriate to seek out a hypnotherapist per se, but rather the services of a licensed physician or clinical psychologist who has training in hypnosis.

It was a German, Anton Mesmer (1734–1815), who discovered a technique which he claimed could produce remarkable changes in behavior. Hypnosis involves suggestion by the hypnotist to produce in the patient an altered state of consciousness that can bring about a change in behavior. This was the original technique used by psychoanalysts (notably Freud) in the treatment of emotional problems. Put simply, hypnotherapy used on its own tries to do what behavioral therapy does: change a learned response (vaginismus) through positive suggestion. The difference is that in hypnosis the suggestion is received in a "trance" state. If my psychoanalyst had used hypnosis, as some do, it would have been as a further aid to the uncovering of repressed material. However, behavioral therapists who use hypnosis (as in Sandra's treatment) do so strictly for the purpose of direct behavior modification or to induce relaxation.

I recommend that hypnosis only be sought from a doctor, clinical psychologist, or qualified psychotherapist or analyst.

JACKIE'S TREATMENT

Twenty-two-year-old Jackie had been married for one year. Because she feared being torn apart during penetration, she had never been able to insert tampons or allow intercourse. She also had a phobia about being vaginally examined. Jackie's GP referred her to a doctor who uses hypnosis as an adjunct to psychosexual skills. The process described here took place over six sessions, each lasting approximately two hours.

Positive Conditioning

In common with other psychosomatic conditions, Jackie's vaginismus was seen by the doctor as the result of poor conditioning deriving from an unconscious block which governed Jackie's reflexes. By putting Jackie under hypnosis, the doctor believed the spasm could be resolved by positive subconscious reconditioning to end the reflex response. If an unresolved emotional conflict has had to be repressed, it usually translates itself into a self-punishing response expressed involuntarily through the body—in this case, the vagina. What the doctor aimed to do was allow Jackie to rearrange the stimulus–response cues which produced her vaginismus.

The Value of Hypnotherapy

Hypnosis allowed the doctor to explore the unconscious reasons for Jackie's vaginismus.

> Not every medical hypnotist uses the analytic exploratory side. Quite a lot will be using hypnosis more as a reprogramming with positive suggestions on the behavioral side, but in the hypnotic trance state where the suggestions are more readily accepted.
>
> —Dr. Anne Mathieson

Jackie found that hypnosis was in itself relaxing and calming. She had inevitably become very tense because of the vaginismus and was able to learn how to induce relaxation in herself. In the hypnotic state, she was more responsive to positive suggestions than when she was wide awake.

> It's not magic. You can't tell a woman, as our fantasies would tell us, to go away, do this, that or the other, but repeated

suggestions in the trance state are more readily accepted. It can be used to suggest a change of attitude and substitute a new way of responding for old.

—Dr. Anne Mathieson

The doctor made general, positive suggestions about Jackie's specialness and abilities in order to strengthen Jackie's ego.

Inducing the Hypnotic State

One definition of the hypnotic trance is that it's a state in which one has shifted one's viewpoint from the rational, logical thought processes of the left frontal lobe of the brain to the more imaginative, intuitive functioning of the right frontal lobe.

—Dr. Anne Mathieson

The hypnotist's method is probably familiar to many of us from TV, films or the stage. However, in reality it is a far more scientific and considered process. The doctor induced the relaxed sensory state (trance) in Jackie in three phases, although—as with any treatment—methods of induction are many and varied:

- Phase One: *eye fixation*. The doctor asked Jackie to focus on a particular object in the room or to close her eyes and relax. During induction, Jackie's attention was fixed when the doctor instructed her to concentrate on the sensation of her closed eyelids.

- Phase Two: *bodily and mental relaxation*. Jackie's doctor asked her to let her mind go along and tune in to what the doctor was suggesting to her. The doctor asked Jackie not to try too hard to concentrate on her every word, lest Jackie become tense and wide awake.

I explain this to the patient as letting her busy-planning-organizing part of her mind freewheel and slip into neutral gear.

—Dr. Anne Mathieson

• Phase Three: *journey into childhood*. Jackie's doctor aimed to find the roots of the vaginismus and Jackie's accompanying anxieties and fears. When Jackie was deeply relaxed the doctor counted down the years, telling Jackie that the index finger of her right hand would lift or wave spontaneously at every year in her life when her unconscious mind was aware of some important root source of fear and anxiety related to her vagina. These years were then explored in turn. The doctor also directed questions to Jackie's unconscious mind, telling her that her right hand would lift spontaneously if the answer from the unconscious mind was "yes" and that her left hand would lift for "no." Once the causes of vaginismus could be traced and identified (not always possible or necessary), the doctor introduced some positive suggestions.

Once one has cleared the trouble, then it's at this point that I might say: "Look, now you can see why your personal 'computer' was wrongly programmed and we must now put in a nice positive feeling if you believe this part of your body is damaged."

—Dr. Anne Mathieson

Contrary to popular belief, at no time during the trance did Jackie receive the command: "When you wake up you won't have vaginismus."

It's not appropriate to tell somebody she won't do something when she still has an unconscious reason for doing it, particularly where there might be a very profound unconscious reason for the spasm. You are then going to set up a great deal of inner conflict which isn't going to be helpful to the endeavor at all.

—Dr. Anne Mathieson

Suggestions to Dissociate Pain from Intercourse

The doctor induced in Jackie sensations of heaviness, warmth and tingling, and in this relaxed sensory state Jackie was open to associative suggestions. These were aimed at inducing in her an acceptance of new ways of interpreting sensations. Since Jackie was acutely phobic about anything entering her, she was encouraged to react to penetration in the context of the nonthreatening, painless, warm and pleasant sensations she was experiencing while in the trance.

> The way I generally put it is to say she will find she has all the confidence in the world and it may well be much sooner than she would have expected it. I also make general suggestions that she will feel more confident and happy about her body, particularly with the sexual part of it.
> —Dr. Anne Mathieson

When this new sensation was sufficiently implanted and Jackie was taken out of trance, her reaction to penetration lacked the usual phobia. However, since Jackie could not live in a permanent hypnotic state or carry the doctor around with her, she was taught to use the technique of auto suggestion, a kind of do-it-yourself relaxation which enabled her, if she ever felt fearful and anxious about a situation, to summon up in her mind the pleasant sensations experienced in hypnosis.

Freud and Hypnosis

The popular image of the hypnotist as a theatrical performer with a swaying watch bears no relation to the serious and committed work of most practitioners. Much of the skepticism and hostility directed toward hypnosis may have been the result of the method's rejection by Freud and the psychoanalytic movement. In Freud's time hypnosis was still in its infancy, and understanding of the process was limited.

Many analysts feared that hypnotists brainwashed their patients, planting ideas in their minds or manipulating them. For a while, Freud experimented with hypnotic suggestion, but he soon found it an imperfect technique, uncertain and often not at all effective. He eventually abandoned the use of suggestion and replaced it with a new method which became known as free association (see "Linda's Treatment," page 154). Although hypnosis does not render a person unconscious, Freud concluded that it could never be as valuable as his method; in analysis patients make decisions and connections in full consciousness, confronting in total awareness the hidden conflicts behind their problems. Accordingly, the majority of psychoanalysts tend to favor free association, believing it a more effective way of reaching a person's unconscious.

Answering the Critics

Because hypnosis is often misunderstood, I asked Dr. Mathieson to clarify specific points with particular regard to the treatment of vaginismus. To avoid any misinterpretation, Dr. Mathieson's answers are quoted directly:

Q: When used purely as behavior modification, does hypnosis work within narrow bounds, since much of the detail of my life is excluded?

A: I always take a very full case history before I proceed with any treatment.

Q: For hypnosis to be effective, is repression of my deeper conflicts necessary?

A: Whatever one does with hypnosis, it's collaboration between patient and doctor, and so long as one has an open understanding between each other, there's no need for repression of any kind.

Q: If I request hypnosis to overcome vaginismus, might I be demonstrating a wish to have it magically hypnotized away by someone else, reflecting an unwillingness to take responsibility for touching my body and being active in the healing process?

A: A woman may well be expressing this wish, but as far as the way I work is concerned she will discover that that's not the way we are going to get there.

Q: Does making problems "vanish" as if in a disappearing act suggest a bypassing of my unconscious?

A: On the contrary, I think hypnosis puts one in touch with the unconscious, and I don't believe one can override the unconscious with simple positive suggestions.

Q: Are the results of hypnotherapy short-lived, limited and artificial?

A: This would only be the case if one was using hypnosis purely to put in positive suggestions. What I aim to do is look at the underlying dynamics, and any changes would be of real depth. However, if one is using hypnosis to persuade someone to do something [she doesn't] really want to do, like give up smoking, then there will be a very high failure rate.

Q: Some of the most damaging criticisms are claims that hypnosis can't be proven. One American researcher says there is no evidence that hypnosis even exists.[4] Is this true?

A: One can prove certain things about the hypnotic state. Body temperature drops and patients start to shiver. If one measures the basal metabolic rate, that has also dropped a bit. In addition, if one obtains electrical brain wave recordings in hypnotic trance, they are different from both the waking and the sleeping state and closely akin to the meditation states.

WHO BENEFITS MOST FROM HYPNOTHERAPY?

Dr. Milton V. Kline, director of the Institute for Research in Hypnosis and Psychotherapy and the International Society for Medical and Psychological Hypnosis, both in New York, confirms that in the mid-1960s the American Medical Association's Council on Mental Health endorsed the use of hypnosis in medicine and psychotherapy. The council indicated that hypnosis had specific value in treating certain conditions, and those findings were essentially the same as the British Medical Association's in 1953 regarding the use of hypnosis to relieve psychosomatic conditions. Since vaginismus is truly psychosomatic, hypnosis may therefore have a valuable role to play in the treatments of some sufferers.

> Hypnosis is an appropriate form of treating vaginismus because one can get down to the roots of what has gone wrong.
> —Dr. Anne Mathieson

If, like Jackie, we are so irrationally frightened of a vaginal examination, hypnosis may deeply relax us and help us overcome this fear. On the surface, hypnosis might seem to appeal mostly to the woman who wishes to be led by a powerful, guiding "parent" who gives her commands. This, however, is not always the case:

> One might play it as the all-powerful doctor making suggestions, but I choose not to do this. The way that I work is that I believe the woman must be responsible for her own life and her own self, and I am there to help her.
> —Dr. Anne Mathieson

PSYCHOTHERAPY

What separates psychotherapy (and psychoanalysis and feminist therapy, which will be discussed next) from any other treatment is its total reliance on the relationship between patient and therapist. When I consult my general practitioner I hope to walk away with the right advice or prescription regardless of whether he and I relate well. The same would be true of the surgeon who may, in some instances, never have conversed with a patient, but nonetheless can perform a successful operation. Because an analyst or therapist does not dispense pills or examine the patient physically, the treatment relies totally on their relationship. This is central to therapy; it is the love★ and security the therapist offers that can ultimately heal, strengthen and make mature the patient's personality.

The need to relate intimately and honestly is what makes psychotherapy the most powerful, yet paradoxically the most difficult, of all methods. A doctor generally relies on medical and scientific knowledge, but therapy requires that the therapist knows himself or herself, as well as the patient as a person. Therapists must be emotionally perceptive and must work intuitively; they must identify with us in order to get to know us. We meet the therapist on an emotional, not intellectual, level, as someone who has faced similar conflicts and gained understanding. The therapist's understanding and knowledge do not come only from theories, but also from an ability to identify and feel with and for the patient.

Psychodynamic technique alone will not cure vaginismus; it is simply a way of investigating the sufferer's unconscious processes, and though an essential part of therapy it is not the healing factor. Change, growth and resolution come about as the direct result of a genuine, loving relationship in

---

★ The kind of love described here is akin to parental love and is known as "agape," as distinct from "eros," which is sexual love.

which the woman is able to discover new knowledge about herself because she feels cared for and understood.

The analyst Donald Winnicott likened the relationship of therapist and patient to that of mother and infant. Just as a mother is free to use both the factual and the personal knowledge she has to meet her baby's needs, so too the therapist will use whatever intellectual knowledge his or her training has provided, but in addition to, not in place of, his or her intimate and intuitive knowledge of the patient.

The term psychotherapy basically describes a conversation between patient and therapist. This method is based on psychoanalytic theory, but differs from traditional analysis in technique, depth, length of treatment and degree of personality change produced.

You may wish to opt for psychotherapy if:

- full-scale psychoanalysis is financially out of the question.
- you do not live in or near a large city where psychoanalysis is available.
- you believe your vaginismus can be resolved without the use of a technique aimed to bring about deep, extensive changes in your personality and functioning.

Psychotherapists generally base their work on Freudian concepts, combining this orientation with aspects of Jungian, Kleinian, Gestalt and feminist therapy (see "Jenny's Treatment," page 168).

MAUREEN'S TREATMENT

At thirty-five, Maureen had been married for ten years and had two children, ages six and two. Since the birth of her second child, Maureen had been unable to allow penetration, as her vagina went into spasm (secondary vaginismus). She told her GP that she had intense pain during penetration, and described to him the traumatic delivery of her last baby.

Maureen's GP examined her but could find no evidence of scarring or any physical reason for the spasm. One of Maureen's friends had recently undergone successful therapy for a psychosomatic condition, and suggested this to Maureen. She contacted a psychotherapist through a recognized organization of trained therapists. The organization's ethical standards required that any therapist treating vaginismus be in contact with the patient's general practitioner, so Maureen's doctor was asked to confirm a clinical diagnosis of vaginismus before psychotherapy began, which he did.

Modified Psychoanalysis Combining Several Techniques

In many ways, psychotherapy is a modified version of classical psychoanalysis. Maureen's therapist tended to be more directive and advisory, as opposed to the traditionally noncommittal, distant analyst. Although Maureen was not required to lie on a couch, some therapists prefer to have their patients do so, as it can help them to focus introspectively. Maureen also had less frequent sessions than a patient in analysis, although again the frequency is determined by a woman's individual needs; and Maureen's therapist tended to focus more on her current life problems, as opposed to her past.

> When I start I always focus on the present situation; then of course in these discussions we try to discover the reason for her fears. The history comes along with the discussion of how she copes with her sexuality.
>
> —Marianne Granö

Maureen's therapist listened to her in a nonjudgmental and accepting way, and the simple act of talking things out had a healing effect. It helped Maureen release anxieties that she had previously held in her unconscious. The holding in of feelings was contributing to Maureen's pain during intercourse.

I tend to pull back from the vaginismus and just say: "Let's get to know you." I explain the process to people that it's a bit like tipping a jigsaw puzzle out on the table and then together trying to see what picture we can get, and the vaginismus would be part of that.

—Jill Curtis

Understanding the Reasons

Maureen's therapy was more concerned with her external life and environment, as opposed to her inner and unconscious worlds, although some therapists work much as psychoanalysts would in this respect. Maureen's therapy aimed to resolve her vaginismus but also gave support to wider objectives, such as improving her life in a general way.

Maureen's therapist did not treat the vaginismus in isolation from other conflicts in Maureen's life, but connected it with the marital crisis she and her husband had been experiencing since the birth of their last baby. Nor was the vaginismus treated directly by examination, reeducation or dilation (as with Sandra, Amy, Louise and Ellen). The emphasis was on resolving Maureen's deeper conflicts, helping her to make sense of the muscle spasm.

I think what makes psychotherapy an appropriate treatment for vaginismus is because you are really going to the roots of something. It takes time, patience and understanding to get to the root of why this particular woman has developed this particular difficulty. You've got to work at it on a conscious level and also on an unconscious level because that's where the spasm is coming from.

—Jill Curtis

WHO BENEFITS MOST FROM PSYCHOTHERAPY?

Any woman unable to tolerate the prospect of vaginal examination or who does not believe vaginismus is simply a sexual problem might find the "talk therapy" more suitable.

However, she would have to be prepared to explore the underlying causes in ways not required of Sandra, Amy, Louise and Ellen. Likewise, a woman who is unable to cope with the more distanced approach of psychoanalysis, who may find it difficult to tolerate having feelings stirred up by deeper probing, or who may be isolated, with little outside support, might benefit more from a psychotherapeutic method, since psychotherapy is generally less exploratory and more overtly supportive than psychoanalysis.

ANALYTICAL PSYCHOTHERAPY, FREUDIAN AND JUNGIAN PSYCHOANALYSIS

As a mode of therapy, psychoanalysis was developed in the late 1890s by Freud and can be considered the prototype of all psychotherapies. To simplify, psychoanalysis consists of two people (analyst and analysand) meeting in order to understand what is going on in the unconscious of one of them. This method differs from most other treatments for vaginismus in that it is not based on the symptom. Ideally, a woman should not go to an analyst specifically for vaginismus, but to seek help in exploring her whole personality.

> If a woman asks for a specific cure, an analyst cannot be tied in this way. Having said this, of course it's true that analysts see people who come to them for all kinds of difficulties, and as part of the analysis the difficulty will clear up.
> —Lorna Guthrie, Jungian analyst

Although I describe psychoanalysis here in stages, it tends not to be carried out in this rigid and precise manner. I also use technical terms to describe the process, but I do so simply to familiarize you with the theories on which this method is based. Let me reassure you that the majority of analysts speak in everyday language and refrain from using jargon. Neither do they force a particular theory on a woman nor attempt to make one fit her psychology. When a woman consults an analyst, the analyst will start where he or she can, and see how the analysis takes shape.

> No well-trained analyst tackles problems head-on in the way that, say, a clinic might. It's a very different approach because there's so much time, it allows for things to emerge in their own way.
>
> —Lorna Guthrie

Naturally, any woman's analysis is considerably more complicated and its journey much more indirect than any simple outline I can show in a few pages. Since every analyst operates within the broadest boundary of possibilities, there can be no typical analysis. Every woman and every analyst are different.

LINDA'S TREATMENT

Analytical psychotherapy is the approach my analyst (a specialist in this method) and I finally employed to help resolve my vaginismus.

When friends discover I'm being analyzed they tend to ask the same questions: "But what really happens? How does it work? Do you lie down on a couch?" Analysis seems to be shrouded in secrecy, so I hope this account will demystify what is essentially a healing process. It may be thought of as repair work, helping to restart the halted processes leading to maturity.

The Need for Further Exploration

Like most people, I knew very little about my unconscious mental processes before I entered analysis. The only person I could think of who'd been in psychoanalysis was Woody Allen. This was as far as my knowledge stretched about the subject. I didn't even realize analysis could help resolve vaginismus.

Although I knew I was suffering from vaginismus and desperately wanted help, I did not know who to approach, so I first went to the obvious people, the gynecologists, as I have already told you. I naturally thought the only way to treat what I thought of as a physical problem would be a physical treatment. It didn't work. Unable to tolerate the internal examinations, I was left feeling overwhelmed and defeated by my condition.

I entered analysis through the back door, meaning it wasn't a conscious decision on my part. In 1981, at the age of thirty and after almost three years of marriage, I made an appointment to see another doctor (my fourth) at a women's health clinic. It so happened that this doctor was an analytical psychotherapist, still practicing psychosexual medicine part-time.

I explained that I'd always felt too small to be penetrated and had an acute phobia about anything entering me. Whenever my husband attempted to penetrate, my vaginal muscles clamped shut and I felt faint and nauseated, sometimes even retching. I described my vagina as a "gaping open wound with bits dangling from inside."

The doctor was able to rule out any physical causes using my medical history (the internal examination described in the last chapter had disclosed that there was nothing physically wrong). His original planned treatment was to counsel me, eventually leading to an internal examination. This psychosomatic approach (as in Tina's treatment) seemed less frightening than my previous encounters with gynecologists, who had always insisted on examining me first. The doctor assured me that he would not force an examination, that it was to be at my instigation and only when I felt ready. However, this was not to be the course events took.

My fears about the internal exam did not decrease over the subsequent weeks, and in the seventh week of therapy I found myself daydreaming about the doctor. It was approaching Christmas, and because of the holidays I was not due to see him for a fortnight. During the break I felt anguished; I missed him and longed to see him. I didn't think I could endure another week, so I telephoned the clinic. On the telephone he suggested I see him in his capacity as an analyst, since a more in-depth therapy now seemed appropriate. I was able to make the transition quite easily from the psychosexual to psychoanalytic setting, since I was still seeing the same person.

Officially, once I'd made the request to see him during my holidays, and had also disclosed the romantic nature of the fantasies I was having about him, my psychosexual treatment had ended. Psychoanalysis had begun.

Repairing Damage

It is impossible to describe exactly what takes place in more than six years' analysis. There were no dramatic insights or theatrical interpretations leading to the instant relief of my vaginismus. Since the roots of the condition lay in my early development, my experiences and relationships during infancy were to be key sources of information for my analyst.

Growth and change are a series of incremental achievements, each slowly building on the other to allow the unlocking of whatever it is the vaginismus seeks to defend. Most of the insights were painful and difficult to reach, since the vaginismus was protecting a multitude of layers, all giving clues to my earliest experience, anxiety and assumptions, as well as my needs and fears. The relationship between a woman and her analyst is always a central theme, because the close, dependent bond tends to mirror the earlier parental one, helping to bring about an understanding and reappraisal of often distorted assumptions we made as a child. Knowing the minimum about my analyst forced me to draw conclusions about things I could not know, thereby giving us the opportunity to re-create feelings and interactions from infancy in the hope that this could lead to a better outcome the second time around.

Growth and change are deemed to be taking place when dynamics such as those I will describe are recognized, identified, understood, separated from the past and, finally, worked through. These are the main routes which can lead to the resolution of conflicts and, ultimately, the reversal of vaginismus.

Free-Flowing Thought

We began by asking ourselves, "What are the conflicts which led to Linda's vaginismus?" My analyst's training taught him that the answer to this question probably lay in the mischanneling of unconscious psychosexual conflicts and an unsatisfactory resolution of the Oedipal complex. To understand how and why this had occurred, he would need to reach the causes buried deep in my subconscious. But how did he attempt to reach that part of my mind whose contents were almost totally inaccessible? He used two techniques.

The first was free association, whereby I said whatever came to mind during a session. This might not seem bold today, but it was an outrageous idea in Freud's time to encourage patients to speak without repressing anything whatsoever. The kind of information important to my analyst was not likely to be gathered by a series of questions like those asked in the normal doctor-patient dialogue. Though answers to specific questions would have provided factual information, this might have been at the expense of a wealth of emotional connections which could only be made if I talked freely and uninhibitedly.[5] Aside from initial history-taking, my analyst asked only the minimum and commented occasionally on what I said.

The second technique was the interpretation of dreams, which my analyst saw as symbolic representations of my unconscious conflicts and repressed erotic wishes.

The other central principles that formed the basis of my analysis are described on the following pages.

Exploration of Infantile Sexuality

Freud believed that we come into the world with our sexual instincts and that at each stage of infantile sexuality, pleasure is obtained from different sexually stimulating ("erotogenic") zones. His general theory was that our libido (sexual drive) in infancy passes through three emotional stages: *oral* (birth to eighteen months), when the baby experiences pleasure from nursing at the breast; *anal* (eighteen months to three years), when the infant experiences pleasure from her bowel movements; and *phallic* or genital (three to four years), when the toddler experiences pleasure from touching her vagina, as in masturbation.

These three stages (and I have only approximated the ages at which they occur) then culminate in the Oedipal phase at age four or five.[6]

The possibility of our becoming arrested at any of these stages in development might affect our behavior in later life. A symptom, therefore, expressed in a particular part of our body may indicate (though never precisely) at what stage of development we became stuck or fixated. For example, oral fixation might appear as anorexia, while a genital fixation might show itself in vaginismus.* So the fact that my spasm was located in my vagina gave my analyst clues as to which unconscious forces were active. In other words, my repressed conflicts were of an intimate nature, probably occurring around the phallic or genital stage.

> I find a common language that has meaning for this particular person.
>
> —Lorna Guthrie

My analyst and I needed, then, to find a way of translating the language of my vagina into the language of my innermost feelings.

---

* Many analysts after Freud, including my own, maintain that the earlier and the less sophisticated the level on which the disturbance is experienced, the more likely it is that the symptoms will be sexual.

My analyst's aim was to unravel and explore with me the conflicts my vaginismus was expressing—in particular, the blockage caused perhaps by my unresolved Oedipus complex.★ The origins of my vaginismus dated to my infancy, when I felt persecuted by my fantasies, and when I made an important discovery which I was too young—too small —to deal with: I saw that adults were able sexually to give each other things that I could not. As explained in Chapter Three, my fear in adulthood of being "too small" to accommodate an erect penis was perhaps another way of saying that my needs, desires and unnurtured part of myself made me feel I was too small, too young and too vulnerable.

Reenacting Aspects of Childhood

During our sessions I lay on a couch so that my analyst and I would not distract one another and so that I would be encouraged to focus on myself rather than on him. The emphasis was more on underlying conflicts and less on the here and now. Our sessions lasted fifty minutes. Insistence on the analytic hour and regularity of sessions also gave me a sense of security and consistency, themes which felt internally absent.

Treatment was intensive, frequent and lengthy (three times a week since 1981 and still continuing). This allowed me to "regress" (return to my infantile and primitive states), repeating and reenacting with my analyst earlier unresolved relationships. This sometimes took the form of experiencing him as the "bad mother," who was tantalizing, powerful and withholding, or alternatively the "good mother," who nurtured, loved, held and fed me psychologically. If I was able to enjoy a satisfying, intimate relationship with my analyst, the persecutory images I carried around inside could be expected to lose their emotional charge.

★ Many analysts after Freud regard the period when baby is totally dependent, not the Oedipal phase, as the stage when psychological problems may occur in development.

Interpretation Leading to Insights

When my analyst made conscious what was emerging in my unconscious, this was called an interpretation. An insight was my capacity to understand my own, or someone else's, mental processes, as well as my sudden understanding of a complex situation or problem. However, in real life, realizations and insights may come suddenly in one session and disappear in another, only to return several months later. This made my progress seem patchy, slow and frustrating, not at all as orderly as it seems in this outline.

One of my analyst's principal tasks was to point out connections between the current vaginismus and events which may have led to it. This included helping me to identify and map out the nature of my emotional processes—for example, why I felt and fantasized the way I did, and the subsequent assumptions I made. As analysis progressed I became increasingly able to make interpretations and connections myself with minimum assistance from my analyst.

> The more a woman knows about herself and about being able to link some things from the past and therefore able to be free of some of those things, then the more she is able to make wiser choices in her life.
>
> —Lorna Guthrie

Other interpretations included our discovery that the muscle spasm was not at the level of my vagina but rather in the areas of love, intimacy, dependence and trust. This was significant, since it meant the vaginismus would not need to exist in my body if I could locate the areas in which it truly existed.

Helping me to understand myself better, my analyst drew to my attention that the way I talked about "the spasm" or "the vaginismus" indicated a natural attempt to distance and separate myself from my difficulty. In other words, I wished to avoid the pain and anguish of seeing the vaginismus as mine, as the angry, hurt and outraged parts of myself.

Repression

Most psychological traumas of childhood are repressed in order to protect us from pain; this means the traumas are pushed into our unconscious or kept from becoming conscious. Thoughts and impulses are also repressed if we feel they conflict with conventional ways of behaving and thinking.

Resistance

Internal conflicts about inner changes, happiness and success were reflected in the relationship between me and my analyst. This is called resistance, and in my case it usually took the form of my not complying with analytic rules (refusing to use the couch, or asking my analyst personal questions about himself and his life).

Resistance was also a defense against my taking in of his undesirable and painful interpretations, which I experienced as a kind of analytic penetration. However, he never accused me of using resistance or defenses intentionally to block him or my treatment. Rather, he saw the appearance of a defense as an opportunity for us to work through remaining areas of difficulty and conflict.

The Past Coming Alive in the Present

Feelings of curiosity, envy and exclusion with regard to my analyst's sex life and lover emerged during analysis. I was re-creating an earlier scenario which came alive as the result of my regressing. Therapy revealed that it was possible that as a baby I had accidentally witnessed or had imagined my parents' lovemaking. Reliving this early experience allowed me to explore buried emotions and assumptions, which resulted from my feelings about the primal scene. I discovered that as a baby I had felt envious and excluded, ashamed and guilty, just as I now felt toward my analyst and my friends. Such negative feelings had led to the assumption that I was wicked, too small and neither woman enough nor desirable enough ever to be lovingly penetrated. I saw that the themes were strikingly familiar: the exclusion I felt then as a baby and how I felt later as an adult when confronted with (or imagining) other people's lovemaking. Before this discovery I often got the sequence of events in the wrong order. I would insist that the vaginismus existed *before* my feelings of outrage toward sexual women. In actual fact, the erroneous assumptions I made about myself had arisen from the exclusion, rivalry, guilt and envy which had led to the vaginismus, not the other way around. Rearranging the sequence of events led to recognition and relief that I was not born with vaginismus but had developed it as the result of intense emotions which I was too immature to cope with.

Loving and Hating the Analyst

Much emphasis was placed on the relationship between me and my analyst, in particular my feelings toward him (transference). Used loosely, transference refers to the flow between any two people in everyday life. This consists of our unspoken attitudes, images, ideas, perceptions and mutual feelings of love and hate. But when I use the term "transference" in connection with my analysis, it refers not only to conscious and unconscious feelings and reactions toward my analyst, but also to those moments when I unconsciously react to him as if he is an important figure from my psychological past (mother or father).

Through the analysis of this transference I wrestled with my past coming alive in the present, and so enabled us to trace these emotions to infantile anxieties. I was not simply remembering painful, repressed experiences, but was re-creating and reliving them, too. Resolution of transference is seen to be critical to a successful outcome because transference mirrors an Oedipal situation.

People make jokes about patients falling in love with their analysts, making it seem a laughable and even trivial occurrence. The intensity of feelings a woman might have for her analyst can be more easily understood if we see what he represents in her life. My analyst assumed great importance because he always believed in my worth, autonomy and specialness, as well as my right to have his undivided attention and to be taken seriously. The analytic encounter was the first time many of these needs had been acknowledged or met. Feelings are never acted on between a woman and her analyst, but they are explored. It is precisely this degree of exploration which distinguishes the analytic relationship from any other that a woman will have in her life.

Loving and Hating the Patient

Now we turn to the analyst, for he, too, experiences emotions.

The term "countertransference" refers to the analyst's feelings about and reactions toward the patient.

> It isn't only the woman who is being explored . . . the analyst is also constantly exploring his own psyche.
>
> —Lorna Guthrie

Because he had been analyzed (a prerequisite for any analytic training), my analyst was less apt to develop countertransference. When it did occur he was better able to understand it, which helped him avoid complicating my own problems. If his countertransference had not been understood by him and analyzed, it could have distorted his perceptions of me and caused him to act in a manner which might not have been in my best interests.

In the course of his own analysis, he had become aware of

his own conflicts and blind spots, and this helped him avoid
reacting automatically to feelings I stirred up in him. If he
had acted on his feelings rather than interpreting or reflecting
on them, it might have led him to play out a role which
duplicated an earlier situation in my life.[7] This kind of scenario played out between analyst and patient, and determined
by the patient's conflicts, is known as a psychodrama.

Interpretation of Conflicts

In contrast with the more directive treatments, my analyst
explored the reasons that I put up defenses of "not knowing"
where my vaginal opening was, rather than trying to
reeducate and reassure me with gynecological diagrams or
self-examination. Rather than appeal to my rationality by
reeducating me when I professed ignorance about the size of
my vagina, he tried to interpret the reasons behind this "ignorance." In the same way, if a doctor had reeducated me
about my anatomy (as both Amy and Ellen were reeducated)
and I had subsequently forgotten what I'd been taught, my
forgetting would have been analyzed as a dramatic demon-
stration of repressive forces at work.[8]

My inability to allow penetration was also not taken literally with the response of attempting to stretch my vagina,
but rather was seen by my analyst as symbolic of my inability
to accept and receive penetrative (loving) interpretations. My
analyst refrained from behaving in a direct, friendly or angry
manner. His professional detachment, as opposed to constant
reassurance, advice and sympathy, was maintained in my
interest and not because he didn't feel warmth or empathy
toward me. The unique experience he offered me by pre-
serving a neutral attitude was that he understood how I was
feeling, accepted it, and helped me to understand and work
through it myself.[9]

Wider Objectives

Success was never measured simply in my ability to allow penile penetration or the disappearance of my vaginismus. Instead, progress was monitored and acknowledged in more profound ways, including my ability to:

- see where the vaginismus is really located.
- identify the origins and roots of my envy and hatred of the sexual and fertile world.
- distinguish my analyst from key (parental) figures.
- notice the past coming alive in the present and how my inner world appears in my outer world.
- own and acknowledge the power of my destructive forces without attacking or blaming myself for needing such defenses.
- symbolize during sessions rather than discuss issues at face value.
- understand the connections between penile and analytic intercourse and recognize that the same protective mechanism is in force as a defense against the stirring up of unresolved incestuous feelings.
- distinguish between subjective experience and reality, between anxiety and fact.
- notice how I take feelings from the past and make them real and concrete for today.
- distinguish a projection (disowning unacceptable feelings and attributing them to my analyst) from reality.
- experience myself as loving and lovable.

Amelioration of the vaginismus which occurred during the course of analysis was regarded as the product of the resolution of my more basic personality problems. We have never referred to the vaginismus as a sexual problem. My analyst saw it only as a symptom about which deeper conflicts were involved, so that it required a deeper insight. Treatment has

not been terminated because the vaginismus has been resolved, but will rather be concluded when my analyst and I
believe the deeper childhood conflicts and transference have
been understood and worked through.

JUNGIAN ANALYSIS

Less commonly referred to as analytical psychology, Jungian
analysis is an in-depth psychotherapy based on concepts very
similar to those of a traditional analysis. This method was
instituted by a Swiss doctor, Carl Gustav Jung, an early associate of Freud from whom he parted in 1913. While the
Freudian may ask, "How did Linda develop vaginismus?",
the Jungian may ask, "What does Linda's vaginismus symbolize?"

A Freudian will probably see vaginismus as *being* the problem, whereas to the Jungian vaginismus can be seen as a
constructive, creative attempt to resolve the conflicts which
led to the condition.

Carl Jung believed that a woman was driven not by sexual
instincts, as Freud believed, but rather by the myths and
symbols of the culture into which she was born. Jung called
this the collective unconscious. To the Jungian a dream would
be seen as symbols, not solely expressing neurotic symptoms
or repressed erotic wishes. So, too, vaginismus might be seen
as the symbol of closed doors, with the doors being closed
from both sides.

WHO BENEFITS MOST FROM PSYCHOANALYSIS?

Those of us who, like me, see vaginismus as part of deeper
emotional conflicts and not merely a spasm of the vagina may
be better suited by a psychoanalytic approach.

Much has been said of the need for articulateness, intelligence and the ability to express one's feelings if analysis is to
be successful. Actually, this is not entirely true. Language

can often be used as a huge intellectual defense, so intelligence does not automatically guarantee success. It could be argued, for example, that a less well educated, less articulate woman might not put up such linguistic resistance.

However, certain aspects of analysis bear consideration. Analysis tends to be a lengthy process, so it is advisable to consider both the financial and emotional commitments before entering into this kind of treatment. As with any therapy, the desire for change is required. Other important factors are a high degree of motivation, a certain ability to step back and observe oneself objectively, the ability to understand symbols, and a willingness to confront painful issues. A woman needs a genuine curiosity about herself and, hardest of all, must be able to tolerate the frustrations inherent in analysis, particularly the painful nongratification of loving feelings. This may sound daunting, but analysis really asks little more of a woman than that she be committed to resolving her vaginismus through the exploration of her psyche.

If quick results are demanded of the therapy, analysis would probably not be recommended. Analysis does not dwell on the symptom, nor does it answer a woman's questions directly. It is far more interested in knowing why the questions are being asked. Asking questions and wanting specific advice were generally seen by my analyst as ways I avoided getting in touch with something deeper and more painful.

FEMINIST PSYCHOTHERAPY

Although we will look at feminist therapy separately, it is not a particular school in the sense that psychoanalysis or humanistic therapies are. Rather, over the years women have involved themselves in many different forms of self-exploration and have created a distinctive therapeutic approach to feminine psychology.

What is specific to feminist therapy—and this is why I believe its inclusion here is valid—is that it is concerned with understanding a woman's internal and external realities together. It recognizes how external events can shape and oppress a woman, at the same time understanding the autonomy and power of her internal world.[10]

The therapy I am about to describe is not exclusively practiced by women, nor is it exclusively sought by feminists. For example, my own analyst was able to explore with me the social and cultural factors specific to my family which may have influenced my psychosexual development. Since feminist therapy does not differ greatly from any mainstream model of psychotherapy, it may be more helpful to read the following not as a separate method but as an adjunct to any psychodynamic approach. I am therefore only describing those aspects which differ, are underplayed or may even be missed in a classical therapy. Jenny's treatment is recounted using the feminist object relations school,* since the term "feminist psychotherapy" does not refer to any one specific orientation.

JENNY'S TREATMENT

Jenny, thirty-four, had been with her partner for four years. Every time her lover tried to enter her during lovemaking, Jenny's vagina went into spasm. She wanted to resolve the vaginismus and was referred to a therapist, who explained to Jenny that they would explore the reasons for Jenny's vaginismus by putting what Jenny saw as her complicated relationship with her mother into a context.

Combining Psychoanalysis with Sociology and Culture

In the majority of psychotherapies, social and psychoanalytic factors are not seen together. Susie Orbach, who has developed (and uses) the feminist object relations theory, told me

---

* As devised and practiced by psychotherapists Luise Eichenbaum and Susie Orbach.

with irony that she is accused by psychoanalysts of being "too sociological" and by sociologists of being "too psychoanalytic."

> For me, these two are absolutely indivisible. A baby comes into the world and is only a set of possibilities. But it enters a social world, and how that world is organized will help her personality to develop. She enters a culture immediately, based upon gender.

How was this approach adapted to Jenny's treatment? Jenny's therapist listened to how Jenny felt and spoke about her relationships with her parents, but in a particular way, ever aware that Jenny's mother's psychopathology needed to be set within a social as well as psychological context. Jenny's hurt and rage over her mother's seeming inability to "be there" for her was acknowledged and took up a great deal of the therapeutic interaction. In time, Jenny came to see her mother's actions as the consequence of the restrictions and demands placed on her. However, it is important to understand that the work of feminist object relations is not about "absolving" the mother. While of course in one sense it is, in another it cannot be. Jenny's therapist recognized the reality of her pain and allowed Jenny that space within her therapy.

> If I hear a woman's pain about her mother not meeting her needs, the way we begin to talk about it will not be to do with Mother's inadequacy solely, but to do with the surrounding circumstances. That's not to deny the pain of the daughter, but to deal with the whole history of generations of mothers and daughters, unconsciously transmitting their agonies. If a mother can't be there for her in a certain way, this is very different from her being wicked or inadequate.
>
> —Susie Orbach

The Difficulties in Becoming and Being a Woman

Because Jenny's therapist had explored and worked through her own pain related to oppression in patriarchy, she was better able to acknowledge and validate the way Jenny had been restricted because of her gender.

> My starting point is how one psychologically *becomes* a woman, and the difficulties that one encounters along the way.
> —Susie Orbach

The imbalance of power in our society, and the cultural norms which demand that girls be sweet and passive and that boys be "out there" and active, frequently prevent women from expressing their anger, hatred and aggression. Since the origins of vaginismus stem from early life, it follows that the nature of the anger and aggression will have a similar primitive intensity. Vaginismus may be a way of voicing anger without having to take responsibility for it and the guilt that follows. However, it can be terrifying for a woman to make contact with the "destructive" aspects of herself which have so long been forbidden, since women are meant to be givers of life, not destroyers. In dealing with this sensitively, the therapist can point out that the suppression and denial of the woman's early distress (feeling powerless or invaded as a baby; not having her needs met) are the reasons that she has been forced to vent this unexpressed anger through her vagina.

The Mother-Daughter Relationship

Jenny saw that one of the reasons her mother had been unable to handle Jenny's distress as a child had to do with the fact that Jenny's mother had not been allowed to have her own distress. Her mother's psychological history made Jenny's distress seem terrifying, making her mother want to silence it. Because Jenny lived in a culture (British) in which psychological distress is not acceptable, the therapist also looked at this aspect of her development.

In Jenny's therapy great emphasis was placed on the relationship between Jenny and her therapist. Together they examined the ways in which their relationship expressed Jenny's terrors, anxieties and desires. Jenny saw that aspects of an earlier relationship were being re-created in the therapeutic setting which had to do with the dynamics between her mother and herself. In the therapy itself, the difficulties with intimacy first experienced in a relationship with a woman were reexperienced, and the defenses against intimacy that Jenny had developed, the attempt to hide her needs and so on, were brought into the open.

> The concentration always on the father feels so wrong for me in relation to most people, be they boys or girls, because *mothers* raise children.
>
> —Susie Orbach

Toward the end of Jenny's therapy, when some resolution, forgiveness and mourning regarding her rage and disappointment surrounding her mother occurred, her mother's own psychosocial position became more apparent to Jenny.

Shifting the Focus from Sex

Rather than seeing Jenny's vaginismus in purely sexual, Freudian terms as the wish to castrate a man or as penis envy, Jenny's therapist encouraged Jenny to make contact with her own symbols and meaning for the vaginismus.

> If a woman describes her vagina as a big gaping hole or wound, my association would be immediately to the lack of contact or love, not the castration complex or penis envy theories. I wouldn't even have thought in sexual terms. If I do think about the penis and vagina, then that would be as

an expression of the attempt to find and express heterosexual love.

—Susie Orbach

Jenny and her therapist worked on their instincts that the vaginismus existed more in the areas of intimacy, love and trust than in Jenny's sexuality or in her vagina.

Vaginismus becomes a defense structure against disappointments in early relationships.

—Susie Orbach

The therapy became a place for the establishment of a new intimate relationship that sought to embrace Jenny's past difficulties and allow her to receive love and nurturing from her therapist, so that Jenny had a secure sense of self, a self that could be open to receiving good things in other relationships . . . and that ultimately could receive a penis.

WHO BENEFITS MOST FROM FEMINIST PSYCHOTHERAPY?

Obviously, a therapy which includes all aspects of a woman's emotional, social and cultural development would be the optimum choice.

A feminist therapist will tend to work in an emancipatory way (that is, using an approach beneficial to a woman's capacity to choose her own way of life). This therapist's role will be to help the vaginismic woman to take a stand on intercourse, whether it is "yes" or "no." Because feminist therapists strive to be aware of their own standards and values, they avoid prescribing them unconsciously to their patients. In this light it is important to challenge the fact that so many therapists deny the body its right to say no to intercourse, because in treatment a woman's struggle to regain the power and control denied her during infancy may often remain hidden beneath the surface.

Not all therapists look at the social aspects of a woman's psychology, although their methods may be sensitive and effective. I hope, though, that there will always be enough individuality in any woman's therapy for her to feel free to discuss and explore all aspects of early relationships, whether the therapist is male or female, feminist or not.

HOMEOPATHY

I have chosen to include homeopathy among treatments for vaginismus because it demonstrates how holistic medicine works, and because homeopathic literature includes far more information on and remedies for vaginismus than traditional medicine.

Derived from the Greek work *hómoios*, meaning "like," homeopathy is the practice of treating like with like; that is, treating vaginismus with a substance diluted many times that produces the same symptom as that displayed by the patient. The founder of homeopathy was a German physician, Dr. Samuel Hahnemann (1755–1843). He was so appalled at the effects of conventional medicine that he was inspired to establish a new comprehensive system of healing. (For an in-depth guide to unorthodox treatments, see *The Encyclopedia of Alternative Health Care* by Kristin Olsen, New York: Pocket Books, 1989 and London: Piatkus Books, 1991.)

VIVIEN'S TREATMENT

Vivien, thirty-two, had been married for five years and had not been able to consummate the relationship, and this had led to the breakdown of her marriage. Vivien's first attempt, at eighteen, to engage in intercourse had been so traumatic that she had developed a phobia about being penetrated. She was referred to a gynecologist, who dilated her vagina under anesthesia. Unfortunately, this procedure compounded Vi-

vien's fantasy that nothing could enter her painlessly unless
she was rendered unconscious. Finally, her sister, who had
recently returned from India, where homeopathy is more
widely practiced, suggested this as an alternative treatment,
and Vivien contacted a practitioner through a recognized
association.

The Three Principles of Homeopathy

The first principle of homeopathy is that a medicine which
produces the symptoms of a disease in someone healthy will
cure that disease in a sufferer. This is what is meant by the
phrase "like cures like."

The second principle is that the more the remedy is diluted
and succussed (that is, the bottle containing the remedy is
shaken vigorously between each dilution; this shaking process, known as succussion, releases the healing power of the
substance) the more effective it becomes. This is known as
potentization. By extreme dilution, the curative properties
are enhanced and all the poisonous or undesirable side effects
are lost. Homeopaths give the minimum dose required to
effect a cure naturally.

The third principle is that remedies are prescribed individually by the study of the whole person, according to the
patient's basic temperament and responses.

Curing the Woman, Not the Condition

The homeopath treated Vivien rather than her vaginismus,
as homeopathy recognizes that the whole body, mind and
spirit are affected when we are sick:

> I don't label the woman "vaginismic" . . . I treat her in total,
> including her emotions. This is what is meant by a "holistic"
> approach.
>
> —Dr. Kenneth Metson, homeopath

In-depth History

The history of Vivien's health since birth was taken in detail by the homeopath, a process that lasted between one and two hours. He looked at her physical, spiritual, emotional and sexual history, carefully recording any traumas and noting her accompanying feelings, anxieties and experiences.

> The history-taking is extensive. I ask about the medical history of parents, her emotional makeup, any traumas which occurred. . . . I ask about her appetite and menstrual cycle. I also ask whether there are any chronic diseases which run through her family. This is not because we can inherit diseases as such, but it's possible to inherit characteristics or susceptibility to ongoing problems.
>
> Dr. Kenneth Metson

Vivien was also asked some rather strange questions, such as did she like thunderstorms, what was her birth like, and did she drink hot or cold drinks? The homeopath concentrated on treating Vivien, not her vaginismus. He did not automatically prescribe a specific remedy for spasm because he believes that women vary in their responses to a symptom according to temperament. Instead, he tried to determine Vivien's unique responses and so was able to prescribe on a more individual basis.

Overcoming Emotional Obstructions

Using a remedy, a homeopath will also seek to trace the origins of a woman's vaginismus:

> If a woman has repressed an emotion into her unconscious, a homeopathic remedy can very often bring this emotion back into her consciousness much as is done in psychoanalysis.
>
> —Dr. Kenneth Metson

However, as with any treatment which seeks to uncover repressed emotional pain, there may be times when a woman's unconscious resistance impedes progress:

Sometimes a remedy will go so far but it just can't quite penetrate the block. In this case I might refer her to a hypnotherapist who uses psychoanalysis. Very often he is able to reach the block and then refers her back to me and treatment progresses.

Dr. Kenneth Metson

Stimulation of the Body's Healing Power

Most conventional treatments take the view that vaginismus is a direct manifestation of an emotional conflict. Homeopathy, however, sees vaginismus as the body's reaction against the emotional conflict as it attempts to overcome it, and the prescribed remedy will seek to stimulate the woman's natural healing responses, rather than suppress any isolated symptoms. In this way, the body is stimulated to react and release its own healing power (as when a cut in the skin often heals with no assistance). A remedy made from natural sources (animal, vegetable or mineral) was finally selected and used to assist Vivien in regaining health by stimulating her body's natural forces of recovery. In Vivien's case, her treatment lasted two to three years; she saw the homeopath generally once a month. At nearly every visit she was given a remedy appropriate for her at that time. Sometimes she noted dramatic changes in her energy and responses, particularly after the first visit, and at other times the changes were subtle.

We are governed by a vital force which makes us tick, think and feel. If this vital force is unbalanced in any way it is going to produce a symptom, whether it be physical or emotional. Homeopathic medicine aims to correct the imbalance of the vital force, allowing our body to respond and correct that imbalance to eventually correct the vaginismus.

Dr. Kenneth Metson

Rina Nissim is a nurse, author,* feminist health worker and founding member of Dispensaire des Femmes, a wom-

* *Natural Healing in Gynecology* by Rina Nissim (New York: Pandora Press in association with Methuen Inc., 1986).

en's health collective in Geneva, Switzerland. Her extensive experience in working with women and health groups in the United States and Central America has led her to develop a uniquely holistic approach to treating women's ailments. It is because she uses naturopathy and homeopathy combined with feminist counseling that I welcome her contribution:

> With homeopathy there is no remedy for vaginismus, as there is no remedy for colds or asthma, but only remedies for individuals. The choice of the remedy will depend first on the "emotional" or the "mind," then the general symptoms, and then only the local symptoms. Focusing on the spasm is not the best way to use homeopathy. I really believe nothing can replace a discussion on sexuality: all the rest is an accessory. Homeopathic treatments depend on the requirements of each individual woman.

WHO BENEFITS MOST FROM HOMEOPATHY?

Homeopathically, vaginismus is not seen in isolation; freedom from the symptom and realizing the full potential of the woman become the ultimate goals. Ideally, all treatments for vaginismus should follow this "whole person" approach, rather than look at the separate parts of a woman's body. Homeopathy also attempts to intervene as little as possible by promoting the body's natural healing powers. It does not call on surgery, drugs or other devices:

> If a woman with vaginismus wants to be treated without the use of surgery, drugs or mechanical instruments, then she should consider homeopathy.
>
> —Dr. Kenneth Metson

However, as Dr. Metson explains, because homeopathic medicine is still not as widely known or available as conventional medicine, he tends to treat patients who have not responded to other traditional methods:

Women with vaginismus often come to me as the last resort, having tried the conventional treatments. Because I treat her, not spasm, I think that's where homeopathy scores.

Homeopathy appeals most to the woman who wants not only to resolve vaginismus but also to improve her health on every level. Since it is gentle, natural and unintrusive, homeopathy can be used in conjunction with any other therapy of her choice. This could be taken as a symbolic expression of a woman's openness, trust and willingness to be supported by several methods in healing vaginismus. Often a newfound interest in regaining full health may lead a woman to investigate alternative ways of living, such as eating a more nutritious diet or taking up Yoga classes, massage or other gentle forms of body work★ and relaxation.

SURGERY

I feel ambivalent about even mentioning surgery, since I do not consider it an appropriate treatment for vaginismus. However, I decided it belonged somewhere in this section simply because women have unfortunately been operated on for vaginismus in the past, and they still may be misled into believing surgery is an appropriate way of resolving vaginismus.

I find it difficult to believe that surgery would ever seriously be considered an appropriate method of resolving a psychosomatic condition. Furthermore, in the context of the con-

---

★ Working on the body can encourage direct expression of emotion through verbal and bodily means, and can increase a vaginismic woman's emotional awareness, particularly if she focuses on her vaginal area. Many women find this through dance, massage, yoga, t'ai chi ch'uan, the Alexander Technique, Reichian therapy or acupuncture. Guided imagery of the body and meditation exercises can also help release the trauma and "memory" which lives in the body. For a complete description of body work and suggestions for exploring the vagina, read Chapter 5, "Letting the Body Speak," in *In Our Own Hands*, by Sheila Ernst and Lucy Goodison (see Suggested Reading).

temporary woman's assertion of control over her own body, surgery for vaginismus seems an anachronism.

What Does Surgery Involve?

Suggested treatments for vaginismus in the 1800s were always surgical, and gynecologists often performed operations on women without consulting a psychiatrist.[11] (See also "Vaginismus in Literature, Chapter Two, page 18.) This is mainly because psychotherapy was nonexistent, and until the advent of Freud the notion of talking through an emotional problem to resolve a symptom was unheard of. Basically, there are two physical procedures which doctors have used to resolve vaginal spasm: mechanical therapy, in which a woman's vagina is widened and stretched (dilated) by a doctor with the help of a speculum or digital (finger) examination; and surgical treatment, which involves far more drastic intervention. An instrument is used to clip off the hymen, and a vertical incision is made on each side of the vaginal opening. The stitches cross from side to side and the vulva is thus widened. A slender cylindrical instrument (called a "vaginal bougie") is then inserted into the vagina to dilate it.

Why Are Physical Methods Employed?

The reason given for using mechanical therapy is that the doctor (as a figure of authority) is giving the woman permission to have intercourse by physically intervening. However, Prof. Dr. Herman Musaph, a Dutch psychiatrist and psychoanalyst who specializes in vaginismus, reports that this technique hardly ever produces results. He argues that if this theory of "permission" is correct, the same result could be achieved simply by talking with the woman and helping her to accept her sexuality and its functions. He further adds that the disadvantage of dilation is the denial of unconscious infantile conflicts which led to the vaginismus in the first place. He points out that using this kind of educational, rational approach may actually thwart the explorative psychotherapeutic treatment.[12] A consultant surgeon in obstetrics and gynecology at a London teaching hospital confirms that dilation of the vagina under anesthetic is never successful in reversing psychological vaginismus.

What is the reasoning behind surgery? The explanation often given is that if the vaginal opening is widened forcefully, vaginismus can no longer occur. While this is correct in that the woman's body can no longer go into spasm, psychologically the spasm can still occur. Furthermore, the last link of the psychological process which caused the vaginismus has been tampered with, preventing psychotherapeutic reversal.[13]

One of the reasons that surgery has been suggested or performed is that vaginismus has been mistakenly diagnosed by doctors as an impenetrable hymen. As a result of this clinical confusion, the hymen has been surgically removed, but such surgery does not effect a cure.[14] Psychiatrist Dr. Helen Singer Kaplan warns that despite being anatomically successful, the use of surgery gives rise to adverse reactions and problems of sufficient severity to discourage its use.[15]

Why Surgery Is Inappropriate

The weight of opinion today is firmly opposed to the use of surgery as a treatment for vaginismus. Prof. Dr. Musaph has written that over the years he has seen many vaginismic women who underwent surgery yet still had spasms of the thighs or anus, just as before the operation. In others, he observed even more serious aftereffects such as inability to achieve orgasm, frigidity and an aversion to intercourse—all problems not generally common to women with vaginismus. It was not difficult for the doctor to link these symptoms with the surgery the women had undergone. He considered the new problems they experienced to be a shift of symptoms, one of the most striking being hypersensitivity of the whole vulva, strongest at the vaginal entrance, making efforts at intercourse torture for the woman. He strongly advises that surgery never be performed for vaginismus, since it reduces the possibilities for successful psychotherapy.[16]

Such a view is also expressed by Dr. Katharine Draper, who has said that it is more difficult to treat a woman who has had surgery or mechanical dilation "because you are just pushing the dilators in against her prevailing fantasies." Dr. Draper adds:

> A lot of gynecologists are still treating vaginismus surgically, but in our studies we found not a single woman needed operating on. A spasm is due to the ideas behind it, it's not a physical thing that you can cut away at. One should try to get to the ideas . . . what it is she is protecting.

As well as causing a shift in the location of the spasm rather than its reversal, surgery has other psychological side effects. Any gynecological procedure performed under anesthesia may be charged with fantasy-meaning for a vaginismic woman, so it is crucial that the emotional implications be discussed. This is so that any unconscious conflicts can be understood rather than acted on.[17] I say this because in some instances it will be the woman who requests surgery and not the doctor:

> I think that the times when a patient has been referred to me with a suggestion that surgery might be necessary, the request has usually originally come from the woman herself who has built up the belief that her vagina is indeed physically too small.
>
> —Susan Tuck, consultant gynecologist and obstetrician

Dr. Leonard Friedman's 1962 book *Virgin Wives* points out that in performing surgery to stretch the vagina, a doctor might even be unconsciously colluding with the patient in considering her vaginismus as purely physical. As we've already seen, many vaginismic women share the fantasy that their vaginas are too small or deformed, which has no basis in fact. What effect might it have on a woman and her therapy if the surgeon shows by his actions that he shares her fantasy, and tries to enlarge her vagina by means of an operation?[18]

In Chapter Three I described the stages in psychological development which particularly relate to the onset of vaginismus. What if, during the course of therapy, a woman gets in touch with feelings of unconscious anger or envy toward men (penis envy or castration complex) or toward the doctor? Could she not then perceive the subsequent surgery as retaliation and punishment by the male therapist for having such fantasies in the first place?[19]

Virgin Wives also reports that the doctor is at risk of acting out a woman's unexpressed fantasy of being raped if he stretches her vagina under anesthesia. This is confirmed after some women awaken from the operation to exclaim how lovely "it" had been, and how much they'd enjoyed "it." This was understood to be a woman alluding to her unconscious wish that her first intercourse be rape, especially if she has always had an irrational fear of pain. Because of the surgery she has been allowed to act this fantasy out with the doctor in that he painlessly "rapes" her while she is anesthetized.[20] Certainly, these aspects of surgery all demonstrate the need to help women understand themselves better through their fantasies, not to encourage them to act on them.

The Therapists' Views

Without exception, all the practitioners I met who treat vaginismus were appalled to learn that surgery was still being suggested or performed. One doctor, in seeking to understand and explain why surgery is performed, suggested that perhaps the gynecologist feels so powerless he has got to do something forceful. Another doctor further explained that because medicine has become successful at doing so many things over the past three decades, many surgeons believe they must do something to make a woman better, and feel helpless if they can't.

To some, the surgeon's knife as a treatment for vaginismus represented a kind of attack on the sufferer:

> I think it's barbaric and is the equivalent of doing female circumcision.
> —Dr. Paul Brown

> It's horrific . . . the woman must feel she is about to be attacked, but instead of a penis it will be a knife.
> —Jill Curtis

Practitioners in the United States are unanimous in their attitude toward surgery as a treatment for vaginismus:

> We are opposed to the use of surgery except in the rare instances of a very thick, tight hymen. Even then, dilators may be preferable because they do not cause yet another sensitizing trauma to the vaginal entrance.
> —Dr. Philip Sarrel,
> writing in "Dyspareunia and Vaginismus"

> The residual of the hymen is only removed in those cases with an established diagnosis of hymeneal syndrome.
> —Dr. William H. Masters,
> Masters & Johnson Institute

> I don't think it's a particularly common procedure in the U.S. In fact, I don't even think it's done at our hospital. I have seen fewer than ten women who've had such surgery. However, the removal of the hymen was often done by a private gynecologist before the woman was seen at our hospital.
> —Dr. Marian E. Dunn

Jill Curtis adds that women's raised consciousness today means not having to accept operations like this any more, and seeing that there are other ways of being treated:

Women's bodies are belonging to themselves now, and I'd like to think this book will help them bolt out the door if surgery is suggested for vaginismus.

Swedish sexual psychotherapist Marianne Granö expresses a similar view with regard to women's ownership of their bodies:

> Because of masturbation and the use of tampons, more and more girls are taking their own hymens, so it's no longer in the hands of the man or the surgeon.

Surgery is inappropriate for vaginismus. An operation performed on the vagina remains an option only for a woman who was born without a vagina or whose vagina has been narrowed by cancer surgery.

DRUGS, TRANQUILIZERS AND BIOFEEDBACK

My disapproval of surgery for vaginismus is followed closely by my dislike of other invasive methods such as:

- Valium—This tranquilizer is used intravenously to break the vicious cycle of fear-spasm-fear-spasm. The choice of tranquilizer is generally determined by the way a woman feels. If her vaginismus is secondary, Valium may be appropriate, but if the vaginismus is caused by a repressed anxiety, which needs to be made conscious, the use of Valium would be inappropriate, since it would only suppress the anxiety.

- Narcotics—A narcotic (from the Greek *narke*, meaning "numbness") is a drug (such as opium or morphine) which can be used if the therapist cannot achieve the desired result. This is known as narcoanalysis, that is, facilitating in the woman an "acting out" by means of a chemically decreased level of consciousness. Generally a

drug such as Methohexitone Sodium is injected intravenously to trace trauma or combat strong psychic
tension.

- Barbiturates—These are sedatives such as Librium or
  Valium, taken orally before attempting intercourse to
  decrease anxiety and muscle tension.

- Biofeedback—This technique involves using a set of
  graded electromagnetic probes as an aid to learning muscle control.

While all the above are suggested as adjuncts to therapy,
their invasive nature and the very real possibility of side effects
do not seem synonymous with a natural process aimed at
helping women understand themselves better.

WILL OUR PARTNER BE INVOLVED
IN THE TREATMENT?

You already know which of the treatments for vaginismus involve the woman's partner and which do not. It might be
helpful to understand the reasons that a partner is or is not
brought into therapy. Of course, there are no set rules about
this, and two therapists of similar orientation may have differing views on the value of a partner's participation in therapy.

Our partners are already involved, since a lover rarely remains untouched by a woman's vaginismus. However, the
extent to which the partner is involved in treatment depends
on the way vaginismus is interpreted. For example, it is stan-
dard practice in Masters and Johnson's approach to treat couples together, since the doctors firmly believe that vaginismus
is the product of a couple's disturbed interactions, with both
contributing to the disorder. While this may be true of some
sexual problems, I find it difficult to see how a man can be
the cause of his partner's vaginismus if she had the condition
before meeting him, or before any sexual activity.

The Partner in Therapy

Some therapists always involve a partner in treatment:

> Right from the word go he is always present.
> —Dr. Paul Brown

However, although the woman's partner is required to be involved in treatment, this does not necessarily imply that he has sexual difficulties unrelated to the vaginismus. Dr. Brown explains his reasons for involving the man:

> There is a difficulty which I've seen in some men that at the point of wanting to introduce an erection in his partner he has become sensitized and rather clumsy due to previous failures. Some work sometimes has to go on with him.

Marianne Granö also expresses concern for the partner:

> A partner must have some support. When a man has been waiting for his lover for years and she starts suddenly to want something, often he can be impotent. What they are doing in Holland★ is that when they begin group therapy for vaginismic women, they also start a group for the partners.

Other therapists involve the partner at different stages, not requiring him to be present at every session:

> I prefer to see the couple together initially. I can observe what their relationship is like and allow them to talk. It's generally quite apparent then which is the more dominant person.
> —Barbara Lamb

As explained, therapy should never be rigid and should allow for individual requirements. Sex therapist Dr. Martin Cole illustrates this flexibility when speaking about the partner:

★ See page 201, "Vaginismic Women's Group with Parallel Partners Group."

Sometimes I involve the partner, but not always. We have a kind of round-table discussion where we work out what the woman wants.

Marianne Granö shares this view:

I don't insist on involving him, though I would ask why she comes alone. If she says that her lover isn't interested, *then* I get interested and ask him to come for one or two sessions.

Dr. Robina Thexton of the Institute of Psychosexual Medicine agrees:

Although sometimes the partner is involved, I wouldn't think of it initially. I would listen to what the woman says about him without needing to see him myself. If he seems to have a problem in his own right, then I would find him help somewhere.

If the program is group therapy for couples, it goes without saying that the woman will attend with her partner. As you will see when we talk about a vaginismus group, the partner may be brought in later if additional problems seem to be impeding progress.

Therapies Not Involving the Partner

Some treatments do not involve the partner because they work strictly on an individual basis; these would be in the psychotherapeutic and psychoanalytic settings. If other people were brought in, the transference between analyst and patient could be altered and diluted, and the repressed infantile conflicts might not emerge so distinctly.

I wouldn't involve a woman's partner because that isn't the way I work. I might well suggest that he might like to see someone else, because sometimes the partner gets left behind.
—Jill Curtis

Unlike directive behavioral approaches, psychodynamic therapy is confined to a one-to-one setting so that the focus stays on the woman with vaginismus. In some instances she may not even have a partner, but if she does, any information about him and the quality of their relationship will come from the woman. Vaginismus is seen as part of a woman's emotional conflicts, the origins of which have nothing to do with her current sexual partner.

Of course, she may have unconscious reasons for choosing to be with him, and she may transfer her unresolved conflicts onto this partner or previous partners, but a psychoanalyst would not see the partner as the key figure in her life, concentrating instead on figures from her past.

The psychodynamic approach seeks to help a woman understand her unconscious choice of partners. Once she understands her responses, recognizes that they stem from unresolved conflicts, and is able to work through any remaining difficulties, the need to remain in an unhappy relationship or exhibit the vaginismic condition will no longer be strong. The analyst will be concerned with trying to ease the vaginismus until its strength dissolves because it is no longer needed. Resolution will include investigating and working through the painful conflicts that the woman has had to repress, but this would represent an attempt to end the psychological conditions that gave rise to the vaginismus, not an attempt either to alter or support the partner.

WORKING IN GROUPS

Vaginismus can also be treated in a controlled group setting, generally with more than one therapist.

GROUP ANALYTIC THERAPY FOR COUPLES

Deriving from psychoanalysis, group therapy was originally designed to make therapy more widely available, and allows for emotional problems to be played out and worked through in a small group rather than individually. Simple group therapy brings together eight or so people. The other method, aimed at treating marital and sexual problems (including vaginismus), is known as couples group therapy.

DIANE AND TIM'S TREATMENT

Diane, twenty-eight, had lived with Tim, twenty-nine, for two years. She had never been able to insert tampons and believed her vagina must be abnormally small or deformed. Consequently, she had always anticipated pain during intercourse and had never been able to tolerate penetration. She had begun to see a sex therapist but had stopped treatment about a year ago, as she didn't believe it was helping her. She felt isolated and wanted to talk about her vaginismus with other people, and she and Tim decided on a couples group.

The Group as a Mirror of Everyday Relationships

Diane and Tim's group was considered therapeutically valuable because, like other well-selected therapy groups, it mirrored family and society. Any unconscious conflicts in the members shaped their behavior in the group, and with the therapist's help everyone began to understand these connections. Diane and Tim were encouraged to express their thoughts and feelings so that the group members could respond. Everyone was encouraged to discuss, interpret, empathize and sometimes challenge what was said. The aim was for the couples to see themselves and their problems more objectively, through the responses of others, and therefore to reconcile themselves to what they really were so that they might become less anxious. The therapist who conducted the group did so in the same style he or she would use to conduct individual therapy, and so depending on orientation and personality the therapist could be expected to be detached, involved or challenging.

Supporting and Being Supported

One of the benefits of Diane and Tim's group was the opportunity for them to communicate their feelings in safety with more than one person. Diane and Tim were told that although there might not be another woman in the group experiencing the same degree of vaginismus, some other female members would almost always understand, since everyone had usually experienced something similar, if less troubling. Though the focus only occasionally moved to Diane's vaginismus, a good deal of time was devoted to sexual difficulties in general.

> I don't usually explore the details of the sexual symptomology in great detail, because it makes little difference to what I do, or to the result. However, people do report out of the blue that their difficulty has disappeared. The fact that they mention the problem in the group seems to lead to a resolution of the problem without any actual discussion of it.
> —Dr. Robin Skynner, group therapist

Couples Group Therapy for a Specific Type of Vaginismus

> In the couples groups we've had many couples with extreme degrees of sexual difficulty, which I'm pretty sure included vaginismus. They've complained of inability to bear penetration, so I've little doubt that the muscular spasm was there.
> —Dr. Robin Skynner

People with certain sexual difficulties reportedly do very well in a group such as the one Diane and Tim were members of. As long as there are accompanying personality problems or sexual inhibitions related to the vaginismus, this type of group is appropriate. However, if the vaginal spasm is more specific, localized or due to a trauma, the woman may find the more direct methods (behavioral and sex therapies) more appropriate.

> I have never tried it, but my experience suggests that an extremely powerful form of therapy for vaginismus with the more straightforward cases would be in a group of women who all suffer from that symptom, led by someone with a good understanding of it.
>
> —Dr. Robin Skynner

Such groups exist, as you will see in "Jo's Treatment," page 193.

Less Individual Attention

Group therapy is less expensive than individual therapy. However, members do not receive as much individual attention from the therapist as they would in a one-to-one setting (such as in Maureen's, Linda's or Jenny's treatments) but there are other advantages, because when a group works well each member has six or eight sources of support and understanding rather than one. It could be that some of us might need different types of therapies at different stages of our lives. In this way it's quite possible for a woman to begin with group work and then gain further insight and the wish to expand by going into individual therapy later.

WHO BENEFITS MOST FROM
COUPLES GROUP THERAPY?

Like Diane, if a woman does not think individual therapy is for her, a couples group might be the starting place for an exploration of hidden conflicts. It should be recognized that a couples group may only be appropriate and effective for the woman whose vaginismus is part of a larger personality problem, as opposed to a more straightforward case, which might be well suited by behavioral therapy. But if a woman is particularly anxious about disclosing herself to others, she might do better with the closer, more nurturing relationship an individual therapist offers.

Since the origins of vaginismus frequently lie in the area of early intimacy and sexuality, individual therapy seems more appropriate for exploring the difficulties vaginismic women have with the intimate act of intercourse. Vaginismus prevents the ultimate in closeness and trust: the act of penetration. It is possible that the wish to avoid such intimacy, dependence, trust and closeness, all issues that come up in individual therapy, might be an unconscious reason for a woman with vaginismus to choose group therapy.

However, group therapist Dr. Robin Skynner explains, it is unlikely that any woman with vaginismus would choose group therapy as a first option. Usually it is sought after individual treatments have failed:

> In an intimate matter of this kind one would always think of individual sessions, or at least sessions just with the one couple, and that is how I usually begin. But it is fair to say that many cases of severe sexual inhibition, probably including vaginismus, have responded well to couples groups after the failure of a long series of analytic and behavioral individual methods.
>
> —Dr. Robin Skynner

VAGINISMUS GROUP THERAPY

As the result of research carried out in 1980 in England, it was decided that because groups had been successful in treating women's other sexual problems, vaginismus might also be treated in a group situation.[21] Groups tend to be small (four women in each), and the method used is behavioral therapy. In general, two therapists run a vaginismus group, making the diagnosis before the start of treatment. Groups consist of seven weekly sessions lasting one hour.

JO'S TREATMENT

Twenty-five-year-old Jo had been living with her boyfriend for three years. Because she could not insert tampons she believed her vagina was abnormally constructed and consequently feared penetration. During the past two years she had tried two different treatments, but neither had helped her. These failures increased Jo's sense of isolation and inadequacy. After hearing about group therapy on a radio program, she asked her general practitioner to refer her for this type of treatment, as she felt the need of contact and support.

Success in a Group When Other Methods Have Failed

> Usually the women who come are the ones for whom everything else has failed, so the group is the last thing to be tried.
> —Dr. Patricia Gillan, consultant psychologist

Like Jo, many of the women who come to group therapy do so because they have not had success in any other setting. The cotherapists heard some of the reasons that the women had rejected the other methods.

Jo and the group learned in Session One that they would be taught how to relax, how to touch their vaginas and find the clitoris. No touching or self-examination took place in the sessions; these exercises were given as homework.

> We ask them to imagine they are about half an inch high, and are climbing up their thigh . . . what would they find inside their vagina? From their descriptions we get an idea how each woman feels about herself.
> —Dr. Patricia Gillan

Continuing Discussions of Progress

Session Two involved a discussion of homework for Jo and the group; this was a regular procedure throughout all the sessions.

Each woman would know what progress each of the others was making. This is nice because it's a sharing of details.

—Dr. Patricia Gillan

During this session the structure and function of the vagina and the pubococcygeus muscle were discussed and illustrated by slides. PC muscle exercises were suggested throughout the therapy (as they were to Amy and Ellen) to help Jo gain awareness of vaginal control.

We ask the women to try and introduce one finger into their vaginas, and then to increase this to two. We also encourage them to insert tampons.

—Dr. Patricia Gillan

Sessions Three to Five consisted of the women's talking about thoughts and feelings associated with their homework exercises. The group discussion dealt with Jo's emotional and intellectual responses to self-stimulation, and various suggestions were offered regarding rhythm and variety of touch. Jo's group also pretended in an exaggerated way to achieve orgasm, to encourage them in self-abandon.

In Session Six discussion centered on Jo's sharing at home all previous experiences and activities with her partner. It was suggested that Jo and her partner begin in a nonthreatening manner such as nongenital caresses, progressing to finger penetration, then genital caresses and eventually intercourse (as in Amy's treatment). Once Jo was able to insert two fingers in her vagina, she was encouraged to introduce her lover's fingers.

Every woman has her own time factor, and some women take longer to achieve each stage.

—Dr. Patricia Gillan

Jo was encouraged to use fantasies when touching her body, and at this stage the group discussed the homework they were now undertaking with their partners.

Session Seven, the final session, was a review meeting in

which Jo was given the opportunity to discuss at length any doubts or difficulties she was experiencing. If any of the women had been unable to complete the tasks they had been given, they might have been offered individual or couples' sessions once the group had ended.

WHO BENEFITS MOST FROM A VAGINISMUS GROUP?

Reflecting the diversity in personalities and preferences, some women do not do well with the probing exploratory therapies. Equally, others do poorly with a behavioral program that is so rigid it uses dilators and nothing much else. If, like Jo, a woman believes she has exhausted all the other methods, she might find the additional support and encouragement of a group setting more appropriate.

Of course, a woman may select group therapy as her first choice, and not because other methods have been unsuccessful.

As with any group situation, therapists are unable generally to work at a pace that suits each individual. However, this need not be a disadvantage, since if a single member cannot progress to the next stage, this problem will be talked through as part of the group therapy process. Another benefit of the group setting is that it can act as a good motivator. One woman's success in working toward finger penetration inspired Jo and the others, who wanted to achieve this now that they had proof of success. Since Jo had often attended individual sessions without having carried out her homework tasks, she particularly found her supportive group a stimulant in carrying out her tasks and achieving her goals.

SEXUALITY GROUP

This is a structured group of six to eight women meeting for two-hour sessions that last from eight to ten weeks. The women who lead the groups are trained to work from a place of their own vulnerability. In other words, the leader is not seen as the "expert" but rather as one who can empathize with a woman's fear of being abnormal. The aim of a sexuality group is to provide a safe and supportive atmosphere in which women can reveal their feelings. Many women feel unsafe talking about their sexuality, and because of the feeling of competition, it is often difficult for women to support each other. The approach of a sexuality group is affirmative and positive, seeking to counteract the negativity and competitiveness that attend women's sexuality in our culture.

AMANDA'S GROUP

Amanda was twenty-six and living with her parents. She had always had an excessive fear about her vagina, particularly that it felt too small to allow penetration. Amanda had never been able to reveal her vaginismus to anybody, and a series of treatments had not helped her. She heard about the sexuality group through a woman friend.

The Program

Sensitivity, trust and sharing were incorporated into a program which focused on women's sexuality. The accent was on education, to help counteract the lack of information about women's sexuality and the absence of permission to enjoy it. Because Amanda had never been able to talk about her vaginismus before, she found it tremendously healing to be able to speak about it safely in such a group.

> The group setting is very important because the actual process of seeing different anxieties and problems gives a woman a learning experience which is more than in a one-to-one relationship. They realize the cultural implications; that it isn't just the woman with her individual background but it's a much bigger picture.
> —Anne Dickson,
> sexuality and assertiveness trainer and author

Some of the themes explored in Amanda's group throughout its ten weeks were:

- *Self-image and self-esteem*—feeling ambivalent about being a woman and wishing for freedom from the need for approval.

- *Body image*—negativity toward the vagina.

- *Self-exploration*—looking at, touching and drawing the vagina.

- *Masturbation*—exploring the myths surrounding it.

- *Arousal*—understanding what can impede and what can increase enjoyment.

- *The role of fantasy*—exploring erotic imaginings and cultural stereotypes.

- *Orgasm*—removing the goal orientation toward climax and understanding physiological responses.

- *Feelings and emotions*—discovering unresolved past events or relationships.

- *Sexual likes and dislikes*—identifying what is wanted and not wanted.

- *Celebration of womanhood*—removing the competition and criticism centered around a woman's own body and the bodies of other women.

- *Partners*—exploring relationships with past and present lovers.

The Contract

Amanda and the group were asked to say specifically what they wanted from the sessions. This was called a contract.

> I feel very strongly that women shouldn't be told what to do.
> I help them work out what they want for themselves by
> making a list and we then work out the stages to get there.
>
> —Anne Dickson

By expressing what she really wanted from the group,
Amanda made an important step toward taking charge of and
feeling comfortable with her own sexual responses and needs.
Feeling less guilty about such needs changed the way Amanda
looked at other people in terms of asking them to meet those
needs.

Going Back to the Beginning

Amanda revealed her vaginismus and the pain and secrecy
surrounding it to the other women. Although the others had
come to the group for different reasons, they expressed much
empathy with Amanda.

> There's a lot of room in a group to allow a woman to be
> different and yet also to belong.
>
> —Anne Dickson

Amanda's history and experiences were also discussed in the
group.

> One of the most moving things I've ever experienced was
> one vaginismic woman's presentation of her story. She de-
> scribed to us the last five years of her having vaginismus and
> the treatments she'd been through.
>
> —Anne Dickson

The other women also told their personal stories and the
reasons they had come to the group. One of the first things
Amanda did in the exploration of her sexuality was to try
and understand how she had learned to behave the way
she did.

We start off right at the beginning, taking a behavioral approach to the problem. This is a process of talking and looking at the messages we've learned about our bodies and our sexuality.

—Anne Dickson

Learning to Love Our Bodies

The group focused on body image, and each woman was encouraged to explore her vagina at home with the aid of a mirror. Information was given about women's sexual responses, and Amanda learned how the impact of past and present emotions can interfere with sexual activity.

Most women don't understand how anxiety impedes sexual arousal. Because of the pressure to always perform we don't allow ourselves to listen to what's going on with our bodies.

—Anne Dickson

As it did for many of the women in her group, Amanda's vagina remained a negative and very impersonal part of herself. She was encouraged to examine, touch, look at and draw her genitals to help affirm their uniqueness and enable her to become familiar with this part of her anatomy.

Emotions were not seen by the leader as overwhelming or negative; when Amanda or the others wept and expressed anger, this was accepted as part of the learning process.

As the result of emotions experienced in the group, some women decide they want to explore further and seek individual therapy later. However, although we can touch on these issues, therapy is not within the workshop framework.

—Anne Dickson

Celebrating the Inner and Outer Woman

In one of the sessions Amanda and the group undressed and had the opportunity to look at each other in an uncritical and noncompetitive atmosphere.

This for me is a real strike for ancient freedoms when women can look at each other's bodies, regaining that childlike ability to look and accept without judging.

—Anne Dickson

The first two thirds of Amanda's sessions dealt with her needs and her enjoyment of sex for herself. Toward the end of the sessions, she looked at her relationships with men. At this stage the group members were encouraged to bring their partners into discussions in preparation for finishing the sessions.

WHO BENEFITS MOST FROM A SEXUALITY GROUP?

Although a sexuality group cannot be called a treatment in the sense that it is not carried out by a doctor or therapist in a clinical setting, it can nevertheless form a valuable part of a process in helping a woman to own her vagina and the fears and feelings she has about it.

I believe with enough time, support, care, permission and information we can beam a bit of love into that particular muscle to allow a woman with vaginismus to let go.

—Anne Dickson

The lack of control women feel they have over their lives, their social powerlessness and its connection to their low self-esteem and self-image are reasons that coming together in a sexuality group can be a soothing and healing experience. While the self-help approach may not necessarily be compatible with the "expert's" philosophy of treating vaginismus, it nonetheless demonstrates the potential power and creativity women have in overcoming their vaginismus. A sexuality group, therefore, may be more appropriate for the woman who prefers to work outside the conventional expert-led treatments.

VAGINISMIC WOMEN'S GROUP
WITH PARALLEL PARTNERS GROUP

While this type of group is, to my knowledge, unavailable in the United Kingdom or the United States, it nevertheless deserves mention because of its proven success in the Netherlands. By promoting it, I hope to generate an interest among vaginismic women and their partners so that it may one day become more widely available.

Dr. Willeke Bezemer is one Dutch sexologist who runs women-only and men-only groups, each for eleven sessions. The discussions include four main themes:

- a woman's desire to have (or not to have) intercourse, her sexual past, experience and upbringing, as well as her desire to have (or not to have) a baby.

- possible benefits, if any, of having vaginismus. For example, does it conceal her lover's sexual problem; is it a way of avoiding having to tell her partner she doesn't want a baby?

- reeducating women about their sexuality and genitals.

- desensitization exercises to relax the vagina, leading to self-exploration.

In many respects Dr. Bezemer's groups are very similar to those in the United Kingdom. However, the difference is that at the final stages in the sessions, when the women are learning self-exploration the partners of sufferers also share a men-only group in which they discuss the same issues.

POSSIBLE BENEFITS OF
PARALLEL PARTNERS GROUP

Dr. Bezemer finds that for a couple who participate in one of her groups, there is not only an improvement in the sexual relationship but also in the relationship generally. Women also report feeling more relaxed, with higher self-esteem.

One of Dr. Bezemer's more important treatment goals is to achieve harmony in the signals a woman makes with her body, mind and speech; that is, enabling her to say, "Yes, I want penetration, and of course I can" or "No, I don't, and in that case I can't." Dr. Bezemer calls this a "two-sided yes" or a "two-sided no," meaning that the woman has achieved harmony.

SELF-HELP

I also prefer to broaden the meaning of self-help in relation to vaginismus. The human psyche has an early need for an environment which allows the development of the potential to relate intimately, both to the self and to others. To disclose one's self requires a loving and secure environment. If the only experience a baby has of the world is one of unmet needs and isolation, her true self remains concealed. The roots of vaginismus often lie in a woman's early life, when her developing psyche was endangered by failures in her environment or difficulties in separating psychologically from her mother. It is well known that a positive, consistent relationship with a therapist can foster the development of a woman's self toward full sexual and emotional receptivity. This is truly what is meant by self-help.

It is perhaps less well known or less obvious that a positive, sensitive pelvic examination can have therapeutic value for the woman who suffers from vaginismus. I have placed discussions of the pelvic examination and self-exploration in this "Self-Help" section of the chapter because these activities should be carried out only when a woman feels confident and ready, unless there is a gynecological problem which requires investigation.

THE PELVIC EXAMINATION

Some psychotherapists feel strongly that there is no sense in performing vaginal examinations if a woman can neither look at nor touch her own vagina, and as a rule examinations are advised against if she has not dared to look at herself. I am inclined to take a more moderate and compassionate view. I believe a pelvic examination can be a positive step toward reversal of the vaginismus as part of a woman's self-disclosure, even if she cannot yet examine herself. Something inside a sufferer may unconsciously prompt her to seek an examination, perhaps to see whether she is psychically strong enough to cope with a situation that she once had to barricade herself against. In my case, physiological forces (and perhaps unconscious ones) were at play which led me to seek a gynecological consultation.

I was in the latter stages of my therapy when I suddenly had unexplained bleeding. I knew I needed to be checked out, yet dreaded seeking help, since examinations had so traumatized me in the past. After I had discussed it with my therapist, we agreed on a gynecologist we believed would be sensitive.

I am about to describe a personal experience which may not be typical, as my reactions to this internal examination were particularly severe.

As with many women who suffer from vaginismus, during my first few consultations with the gynecologist, he was unable to do more than talk with me and touch the entrance to my vagina with the tip of his finger. However, this experience felt different from my previous encounters with gynecologists. For one thing, my therapy had helped me to develop a stronger sense of self, making me feel more able to cope with any psychic pain which might accompany a pelvic examination. Second, the gynecologist was very receptive to me and my predicament, and was genuinely more concerned with helping to alleviate my suffering than with getting the job done quickly with the least fuss.

On about the fourth consultation I was asked to remove my underpants and lie on the examination table with my knees spread apart and the soles of my feet together. My whole body trembled violently in anticipation of the examination, as though "remembering" something that I was consciously not aware of. The doctor's response was to reassure me that although he regretted the degree of my trauma it was safe for me to shake or even to vomit, and he encouraged me to "go into" my fear instead of turning away. In the same way my analyst had "heard" my pain at our very first meeting, so this gynecologist was "seeing" my pain and allowing me to "go with it." He suggested that I place my hands on the insides of my thighs to try and keep my legs from trembling, and then he held a mirror in front of my vulva and helped me sit up slightly so that I could see. I began to perspire, felt very sick, closed my eyes and turned away. When he made further suggestions I even placed my hands over my ears and eyes, as though it was not just my vagina that was closed but also my hearing and vision. I experienced his verbal communication as if it was the threatening invasion of a penis, and once I understood this, I was able to open my eyes again and look into the mirror.

The first thing he pointed out to me was my labia majora (the outer lips of the vagina), which are covered with pubic hair. The doctor gently parted these to give me a view of the labia minora, or inner lips of the vagina. All the while I was shaking all over, breathing rapidly, and making a tremendous amount of noise. As the labia majora were parted, I could see my clitoris at the top of the inside folds where the outer and inner labia come together. I remarked that my vagina resembled a gaping, bloody wound, and I suddenly felt extremely small and vulnerable and began to cry. The imagery seemed to symbolize all my past and current rejections and hurt, combined with an overwhelming sense of my unlov-

ability. This visual metaphor was as much as I could
felt faint and nauseated and began to retch.

Two weeks later the gynecologist managed to insert one
finger deep into my vagina, through the hymen until it
reached my cervix. It was my first conscious vaginal examination. I sobbed uncontrollably throughout, yet somehow was determined to break through. I had been feeling
extremely depressed and hopeless that day, and because I had
clearly conveyed my desperate desire to be examined at the
outset, the doctor did not feel the need to stop the examination, despite my ambivalent pleas and cries. At times I even
attempted to push him away.

Afterward, I was surprised to find that the emotions the
psychic trauma put me in touch with (wanting to die, fearing
that I would be split in two, longing to be physically held
and loved, and feeling shame and humiliation) were much
harder to bear than anything physical. In fact, I remember
thinking how comparatively painless the physical procedure
had been, yet how costly in emotional terms.

What I gained from this—and subsequent examinations—
was the reassurance that not only did I contain a space which
could be entered and filled, but I could also survive penetration. However, it should be stressed that continuing to push
into the vagina of a woman who believes she has no space
inside may only reinforce more strongly the sense that she
has no vagina.

The following week the doctor encouraged me to insert
my own finger in my vagina. At first I flatly refused, mostly
because of my pervading fantasy that there was no space
inside, and therefore my finger could not be expected to find
the entrance to nowhere, but also because I was unconsciously
groping around for the space to appear inside me.

A sense of having vaginal space may be compared to the
space that is created between two people in order for them
to have any kind of intercourse, including sexual. In everyday
life this space is rarely conscious, but it was most evident in

my therapy when, sometimes, I felt a hesitation on first being in the room with my therapist at the start of a session. I was searching to find a kind of intimacy, love and acceptance with him before I could make my first verbal communication.[22] In the same way, I only felt able to open up vaginally and accept the gynecologist's examining fingers when I felt loved by him. By "loved" I mean accepted and admired, respected and recognized. I needed both my qualities and my flaws to be seen neither as too wonderful nor too overwhelming, but rather appreciated as integral parts of myself. In other words, I needed a space to be me.

Some Advice About the Examination

When you are asked to lie down on the examination table with your knees apart, you will find that your whole pelvic area relaxes if you allow your waist and bottom to drop down heavily onto the table.

I was also encouraged to produce my spasm deliberately, which demonstrated that I had more muscle control than I had imagined. Also, the more the gynecologist "welcomed" my vaginismus, the more I felt this part of me was being accepted. And the more consciously I produced the spasm, the more difficult it was for my muscles to unconsciously contract.

Try to explore with the gynecologist the positions in which you feel most comfortable being examined. Because of the natural childbirth techniques he had developed in his obstetrics practice, my gynecologist was able to suggest alternative examining positions which helped release the muscles of my pelvic floor, thus making it less painful when the spasm involuntarily appeared. These positions derive from ancient yoga postures and were rediscovered* by pregnant women

* These positions were rediscovered by Janet Balaskas, the internationally renowned campaigner for women's rights in childbirth. She is the founder of the International Active Birth Movement and runs the Active & Aquatic Birth Centre in London.

to reduce the pain of labor and ease delivery by going with the force of gravity. They are instinctive—natural yet forgotten—movements which can be practiced daily to help relax and open the pelvis. The first position can also help reduce the pain of menstrual cramps. While these new positions may feel strange at first, they are certainly worth a try, especially if traditional methods do not succeed.

In the first position, you squat on the floor with your feet apart, flat on the floor, and your hands holding the back of a chair for support. The gynecologist can introduce examining fingers from the side or front.

Another position is a variation on the first: you squat on the floor and lean forward onto a chair or cushions. The examination can be comfortably carried out from behind.

In the third position, you sit sideways with your hip touching a wall and swing around so that your legs extend upward with your buttocks touching the wall. You then open your legs wide. This position is most beneficial to vaginismus sufferers since it releases tension from the adductor muscles of the inner thighs, which have a major influence on the vaginal area. Releasing the adductors can help make you feel more open and relax the vagina, allowing the doctor's examining fingers to be introduced from slightly above you.

I was surprised and delighted to discover how much easier it is to be vaginally examined in these ways,* though it may require a degree of innovation and inventiveness on your part and that of your gynecologist.

---

* Different positions may help many vaginismic women during the pelvic examination, and it is important to remember that often cultural bias rather than scientific fact determines certain practices. In her book *Medicine and Culture: Notions of Health and Sickness* (New York: Henry Holt, 1988 and London: Gollancz Paperbacks, 1990), Lynn Payer explains different medical practices around the world. She tells the story of a British physician who took his wife to the American clinic where he was temporarily working to show her the position American women customarily assume for a pelvic examination. The doctor's wife felt that lying on one's back with feet in stirrups was "barbaric." While her husband was ridiculed by other doctors for performing internals with women lying on their sides, he soon found a line of patients outside his office who had heard he examined "the English way."

A Note to Examining Physicians

As explained earlier, vaginismus challenges many unconscious fears and may produce internal conflicts in the doctor confronted with it. Little information is available regarding the transference and countertransference aspects of treating vaginismus with a male gynecologist, and while this needs to be explored further I hope my own experiences offer some suggestions which can generate a more creative partnership between gynecology and the treatment of vaginismus. If a woman presents this book to you, I hope this chapter will create an opportunity for you both to help lessen the trauma of her first pelvic examination.

First, you need to reassure your patient that speedy progress need not be a priority, since every woman goes at her own pace. However, at times it may be appropriate to point out to her that her need to remain passive and go slowly forces you to push things along, and to ask her how this makes her feel. When this was brought to my attention I was able to recognize the regressive and undeveloped aspects of myself I was playing out with the gynecologist: I needed him to mother and spoon-feed me to compensate for my not having had enough of that during infancy. Recognizing that I was no longer a baby—and that the doctor was not my mother—helped me to see how I could risk being less passive, more powerful and ultimately more responsible without fear of attack from an internalized mother. (See "Linda's Treatment," pages 154.)

It is also important to understand that vaginismus originates in the first years of a woman's life, which accounts for the primitive, intense and raw nature of the feelings often aroused in her during the vaginal examinations, which may also surface in her relationship with you.

However, the most important factor which enabled me to undergo full pelvic examinations was the gynecologist's ability to tolerate my fear and panic, anger and hopelessness.

During examinations I felt pain and fear, disgust and rejection, and "pushed" them into the gynecologist in the hope that I would get back love and warmth which would take my pain away and replace it with something good. This is "projection," whereby we put unwanted parts of ourselves into others and take bits of others back into ourselves, and how, as babies, we originally learned the process of intercourse (giving out and taking in). During my infancy my mother would normally have been the container for some of my intolerable fears and feelings, but because the bond between us had been disturbed I had never had a good enough experience of this.

In a sense the gynecologist became my good container during the examinations, because he did not retaliate and therefore showed me he could survive. By "retaliate" I mean he did not try to suppress my anger, make light of my suffering, shout or physically hurt me, as previous doctors had done. He was able to bear my panic as well as tolerate the hopelessness I expressed and the impotence I made him feel whenever the spasm was too strong for him to complete an examination. Not only were my fears of annihilation turned into good feelings, but for the first time I also sensed the existence of a good container: someone out there who could take lumps of my terror and frustration and change them into something bearable, worth having and, perhaps, even enjoyable.[23] I was able to allow examinations simply because the gynecologist could "hold" the pain and destructiveness, the outrage and confusion that the examinations aroused in me and, sometimes, in him.

Finally, at the end of every consultation you and your patient should have the opportunity to discuss your feelings during the examination. You can convey to her that as her container you are neither completely vulnerable nor indestructible; not perfect but usable.[24] Through these consistent exchanges I discovered that the good container inside me was resilient enough to bear panic and fear without splitting apart or being destroyed forever. The annihilation and disintegration I originally feared when being penetrated had been understood and worked through, simply because the gynecologist had been able to "hold" these feelings for me during the vaginal examinations, in the same way my therapist had done in the analytic setting.

SELF–EXAMINATION AND SELF–EXPLORATION

I am frequently asked, "When is the right time to try and examine myself?" and, "Will it help to resolve my vaginismus?" No single answer can apply to each individual, since our symptoms can vary so much. For example:

- Some women can undergo vaginal examinations without any difficulty, can insert tampons and their own fingers, can even receive one or two of their lover's fingers in the vagina during lovemaking, and yet have intense muscular spasms as soon as a penis attempts to penetrate.

- Some women find penetration by a penis, tampon or their own fingers impossible, yet can easily accept their partner's fingers during lovemaking or their gynecologist's fingers during examinations.

- Some women experience a spasm as soon as the gynecologist merely points his finger in the direction of their vagina.

These variables make it impossible to generalize, which indicates that advice should only be offered on an individual basis. First, though, we need to understand exactly what self-exploration means to the woman who suffers from vaginismus.

Exploring the Boundary

Boundaries are where we (our bodies) end and someone else begins. To use a buzzword, they define our personal space. Vaginismus represents the quintessential boundary, because for a vaginismic woman her psychological boundaries are represented by her vagina.

Regrettably, during my early development the process of psychologically separating from my mother did not go as it should, giving rise to a shaky sense of self which forced me to create a false boundary: the vaginismus. My spasm was the bodily solution my psychology sought to protect the only boundary I was sure of—my body (vagina). It was my attempt both to build a sense of self and to prevent merger with my mother, because for me that meant disintegration and loss of self. As I developed I unconsciously grew to perceive sexual intercourse as the penetration of my boundaries, and I feared that if I let go of the false boundary that my vaginismus stood for I would psychically break apart.

Recognizing and having compassion for these unconscious conflicts may make it easier to understand the terror and why it is impossible for many vaginismic women to introduce their own fingers into their vaginas (their boundary). First a sense of self and separateness must be created that feels safe and unimpinged upon.

Re-creating the Boundary

The desire to explore my vagina emerged gradually as a result of having consistently good experiences with a therapist who felt "at one" with my pain: a human being who cared and could "hold" the unintegrated (split) parts of myself. This laid the foundation not only for my much-needed boundaries, but also for a sense of myself as separate yet integrated, safe from invasion.

An unconscious sequence of internal events seems to have

led to my self-exploration. I increasingly felt I was not only lovable but, more importantly, strong enough to withstand failures and come through them. Such feelings enabled me to consult the gynecologist and subsequently to allow him to examine my vagina. In experiencing a sense of genital space I began to be interested in my body and its contours, my femininity and sensuality. I began to believe that my vagina was a good and roomy, warm and welcoming place to be. A space that had previously been nonexistent and lifeless, without sensation or desire, suddenly contained an urge to be touched, entered and filled. It no longer seemed the dark, slimy, minuscule hole I had so often feared and fantasized about. Once I had understood how my early difficulties with separation, invasion and merger had led me to create a false boundary (spasm) as protection, then, and only then, did I feel safe enough to explore my vagina.

However, this still leaves unanswered the questions of whether a woman should examine herself—if so, when, and how will she know she is ready? The notion that we need to be doing something tangible to resolve vaginismus is something I struggled with in therapy. It was as though I had no trust in my natural healing processes, which is understandable given that my early environment had failed me. At times I felt my progress was so slow that I acted on the impulse to test whether the spasm was still strong by trying to examine myself. Invariably the spasm remained strong, because I was not ready. Whenever this happened my therapist would urge: "Whatever it is you're doing, do less," meaning that internal psychological growth is not something we can forcefully make happen. Rather it is a natural process which needs to be allowed and made room for.★ Bulbs you plant in the garden need the right soil and care, but they do not have to be *made* to grow into flowers, because as the bulbs already

★ The ability to "be" with myself rather than "do" was a process which began during my therapy and can be likened to the practice of meditation.

have life in them, it comes naturally.[25] So too with self-exploration. When the time is right, your psyche will let you know.

The following is a guide to self-exploration and was devised by the author with the kind assistance of Dr. Prudence Tunnadine, scientific director, Institute of Psychosexual Medicine, London.

- Choose a quiet space where you feel safe and relaxed. Let yourself discover a position which allows your pelvic area to relax and open up (squatting might be best). Find your vaginal opening with your fingers so that you can "see" the entrance clearly. (You may use a mirror if you wish.) Ask yourself how this makes you feel. If you find any stage difficult, stop and ask, "Why is this difficult?" If you are too fearful to move onto the next stage, do not force yourself, and try not to feel bad about your anxieties. You may be able to try again tomorrow.

- If, on the other hand, you can move on, touch the vaginal entrance gently and then press your finger into the opening. It won't appear as a hole until you press your finger in. Remember, the vagina is a *potential* space. If the muscles immediately go into spasm, pause. A little lubrication may help. Can you go any farther? If you can't, at this point try to "stay with" the spasm. Sometimes purposely tightening and then pushing down helps relax the muscles. If you feel too anxious, stop and try again another time.

- If you can continue, try to push your finger in and bear down a little, as though you're pushing something *out* of your vagina. Leave your fingertip there for a couple of minutes to get used to the sensation. Do you feel any unease so far? If so, try to think about what might be causing it.

- Consciously try to tighten the muscles more, so that you can feel with your finger that the grip is under your control. Your finger will slip in as the muscles open to let it. Know that these muscles are under your control. Just half an inch will do for now. How does it feel? Practice tightening and relaxing this muscle.

- Congratulations! If you've come this far you're doing brilliantly.

- Once you've reached this stage, it should be easy for you to insert your finger as far as it will go. Feel the stretchiness inside your vagina. Now try to insert two and three fingers. Feel around . . . there's enough room to let an erect penis in, or a baby out, without damage. Do you feel any anxiety? Can you think what it's about? If at this stage you feel very frightened and are unable to go on, try not to feel defeated. Know that the nature of vaginismus may make you feel you must struggle and manage alone, and feel despair and shame if you can't. Try to talk through these feelings with a therapist or an understanding gynecologist.

- If you have managed to insert three fingers comfortably you will probably have overcome a lot of your fear of penetration, at least enough to make it possible to attempt intercourse. If you have a partner, take it very gradually, building on the progress you've made so far. Follow the same sequence as above, but this time use your lover's fingers and gradually introduce his penis inside you.

Lovemaking

Although the self-exploration guide ends here, in reality this will for many of us mark the beginning of a full sexual relationship and communication at the deepest level with our partners. Making love after a long period of vaginismus can be a joyously fulfilling, tender and exciting experience. However, it may also bring up much buried hurt, rejection and anger from the past which may need to be addressed, worked through, and finally healed. Always try to remember that in any physical contact between two people there are bound to be occasions when it is problematic, maybe even painful. The ebbs and flows in our sexual desire and energy, coupled with stress or anxiety, can all affect the way we give and receive bodily pleasure.

While the vaginismus may no longer be a part of our lives, the everyday issues of intimacy and interdependence, sexuality, and relating to one another will continue to present challenges as part of the human experience and the potential to expand our trust, creativity and love.

SELF-HELP GROUPS

A self-help group is a beginning, it's not an end. The other women in my group are actively in therapy, but at least they know there are other sufferers.

—Jan,
referring to a self-help group for victims of violence

As outlined in Chapter Four and described fully in this chapter in ''Self-Examination and Self-Exploration'' (pages 210), some women are relieved and delighted if they can accomplish self-examination of their vagina. However, if this kind of self-help is impossible, a woman should never feel she has to struggle alone in resolving vaginismus.

While supportive, valuable and validating, self-help groups

are no substitute for one-to-one or group therapies. Perhaps we should not consider self-help groups as a treatment but rather as a means of integrating longed-for support into a woman's inner world.

> I used to wonder if there was anywhere I could write, though I don't think I'd have had the courage to start my own group. I'd never heard of self-help groups but I would have liked to have met with other sufferers.
>
> —Sarah

Feeling Defeated by Our Failures

Repeated failures at self-help may produce a defeatist attitude in which vaginismus is seen as insoluble or too huge for anybody to deal with. My own experience confirms that some self-help groups may have limited insight and value, simply because each woman is struggling with her own turmoil without any leader or therapist to intervene and guide her.

Struggling Alone Against Powerful Conflicts

Despite the abundance of sex manuals providing instruction and encouragement to enjoy and improve sexual intercourse, there is no firm evidence that they help resolve problems, or that the techniques they set forth are efficient. The conflicts which caused our vaginismus will not yield easily to self-questioning. This is why techniques for self-discovery can only go so far without another person (a therapist) trained specifically to help in an objective way. This is particularly true of vaginismus, whose buried causes a woman may struggle with alone in vain.

Nevertheless, self-help groups have a lot to offer some women. At worst, a woman might find that her specific needs are not being taken into consideration enough, and this might lead her to seek individual and more structured help, using the group simply for support. While a self-help group cannot be seen as a total therapy in itself, the value of bringing women together to talk about their experiences and give mutual support should never be underestimated. This is especially true for women with vaginismus, as it is not easily discussed or understood.

> Suddenly it's like I've come home. All these women are the same as me . . . they can't make love . . . and they are all shouting for help.
>
> —Jan

If you would like to be part of a self-help group I have listed some suggestions in the self-help resource guide in the Appendix.

Resolve: The Vaginismus Support Group

Although support groups for women have rapidly spread throughout the United States and the United Kingdom, which focus on a range of issues (endometriosis, premenstrual syndrome, infertility, positive cervical Pap tests), there has never been a vaginismus support group.

On April 4, 1990, in response to requests from women who contacted me after reading this book, I founded Resolve, the vaginismus support group. At the time of this writing, membership is small but growing, and because the women live long distances apart and are not able at present to meet, they are confined to supporting each other through letters or phone calls. What women find most comforting about Resolve is the fact that they can talk about their painful feelings of shame and isolation, in confidence, with women who will understand. An added bonus is the support that women who have resolved their vaginismus (and have gone on to have children) can offer to members who have yet to break through. For further information about Resolve, see the self-help resources in the Appendix.

HOW WELL DO THE TREATMENTS WORK?

About the only thing we all have in common is the fact that we are all different; and a woman who has vaginismus is as much a unique individual as any other woman. It follows that her response to treatment will vary, too, reflecting her individuality. Statistics, however, do not reflect these differing needs and do not take into account that what works for one woman might not for another.

All sorts of studies claim success in eliminating the phobia of penetration by behavioral therapy, hypnotherapy, sex therapy, psychotherapy and psychoanalysis. This establishes that *any* treatment can be successful in resolving vaginismus so long as the woman believes the therapy is right for her particular needs. Naturally, everyone concerned with treating vaginismus will want a happy outcome, but I do feel that statistics claiming success rates should not be taken as an indicator of what method is best, nor should statistics determine what type of therapy a woman should choose. How is a woman going to feel, for example, if she does not respond well to a method that claims one hundred percent success?

WHICH THERAPY FOR VAGINISMUS— BEHAVIORAL OR PSYCHODYNAMIC?

> I have great faith in psychotherapy . . . but it does take a lot of time.
>
> —Emma

I hope my descriptions of various treatments have shown you the differences between, say, a behavioral and a psychodynamic method of treating vaginismus. If you think of Amy's treatment in comparison with my own, you will see they are quite different.

The striking difference between behavioral and psychodynamic therapies has been cleverly described in Thomas Kiernan's book *Shrinks, Etc*, comparing it to a volatile situation such as firefighting:

> Behavioral therapy sees itself as the fireman who pours water on the fire, while the psychodynamic therapy is the fireman who stands around and discusses how the fire started and what kind of fire it might be before rolling out his hose. Such a pragmatic viewpoint as the behavioral fireman takes may seem beguiling at first glance, but the psychodynamic fireman might respond by saying that turning on the hose before determining whether the fire is a wood or an oil blaze can have disastrous results.[26]

This example demonstrates the divide between the behavioral and psychodynamic approaches to problems. While it's perfectly possible to introduce analytic technique into a behavioral method (as in Ellen's treatment), psychoanalysts generally don't believe that behavioral methods can be integrated into their own. One of the explanations given is that an analyst who is more directive, advisory and active may upset the interflow of unspoken feelings and fantasies between him and his patient. As we saw in "Linda's Treatment," transference is a central issue to be worked through in analysis. Analysts also see behavioral therapy as an incomplete approach; they argue that even if it changes one aspect of behavior, vaginismus is only a small part of the problem embedded in a woman's personality. They add that the limitations of behavioral therapy mean that it often must be combined with counseling, hypnosis or other techniques. In contrast with analysis, much of the richness of detail about a woman's past and psychology is generally not considered in behavioral therapy.

However, behaviorists challenge these criticisms by declaring that the limitations of their method only pose a problem when trying to understand the causes behind vaginismus, and they claim this understanding is not necessary to help most women overcome the condition. Unlike analysts, behaviorists say they promise the woman only relief from vaginismus, not any deeper, lasting personality changes.

Although the different approaches may seem poles apart, in reality most practitioners are eclectic, using and combining each other's methods and respecting each treatment for its own merits:

> I don't think hypnosis is the only road. I feel sure that psychoanalysis is probably a road that will lead there. It may be that one is a very enriched personality at the end of analysis. It may also be that other direct approaches miss out if one tries to produce something too intensive in a woman who has a deeper problem.
>
> —Dr. Anne Mathieson, medical hypnotherapist

THE RESULTS

It is impossible to say categorically that one treatment is better than another because there are no studies or statistics comparing the goals of various methods.

As psychologist Dr. Paul Brown comments:

> I'm a bit hesitant about making comparisons because there hasn't been a good clinical trial of methods. All I know is that we (behaviorists) can help women with vaginismus. The reasons I think this particular approach works is because it's (a) about reducing the fear and (b) about the acquisition of a skill, which is true in all kinds of areas of life.

I have not listed the published success rates of each method; they can be found in the literature, and I do not believe they have any real value. The choice of therapy a woman makes should not be determined by statistics but by her knowledge and instincts.

What Makes for a High Success Rate?

It seems the more careful the selection of sufferers, the more successful (in terms of achieving penetration) the results. "Excellent" results may be achieved with a woman who, despite her vaginismus, is basically healthy and has a good marriage; "poorer" results if there is a serious personality disorder or marital conflict. Masters and Johnson's high success rate (100 percent) has often been attributed to the strict selection of vaginismic women accepted into their treatment program.[27] If a sufferer is chosen whose characteristics (highly motivated, with a stable relationship and no severe psychological problems) make for a successful outcome, that does not prove that the treatment is better than another. The acid test is the question whether this high success rate can be achieved with unselected women. Think of the school which only selects the brightest pupils and then reports outstanding academic results. Does this prove the school is the best, or merely that such a skillful selection of candidates ensures good results?

What is Meant by Success and Failure?

How should we define the "success" of a method which treats vaginismus? Is a treatment deemed successful because the spasm is extinguished, or should it be measured by the way a woman reports she feels—more confident, happier, able to communicate her needs?

Has treatment failed if vaginismus continues but there is marked improvement in a couple's relationship, with renewed closeness and honest communication? Has treatment succeeded if vaginismus is resolved but the woman's lover goes on to experience a sexual problem?

Likewise, has treatment failed if vaginismus is not resolved during therapy, but one year after termination the condition disappears?

I can think of at least two cases of vaginismus where we terminated treatment and then within six months to one year the women telephoned and said, "It's better."
—Dr. Martin Cole

How would this be statistically reported—as a failure or a success? And did therapy play any role in the resolution? If so, what role? Since figures are never what they seem, all these questions need to be asked when looking at the success rates.

Most studies consider successful penetration and intercourse the criteria for successful treatment of vaginismus, but ideally a therapist should have more individual goals for the patient. As I mentioned earlier, Dr. Willeke Bezemer stresses that her aim is to reach harmony in a woman's verbal and bodily expression. That is, body and mind and mouth say, "Yes, I want penetration, and of course I can," or, "No, I don't want penetration, and in that case of course I can't."[28] This puts a very different light on those 100 percent success rates. While that figure tells us that women are allowing penetration, it does not confirm harmony. For example, I felt powerless because my body would not obey my orders . . . I felt it cheated me. I said, "I want penetration," but my body said, "No, I don't want penetration." I also felt that my mouth deceived me, since my body expressed my feelings honestly, whereas my speech did not.[29] It is therefore important that the goal of therapy be to reach a harmonious integration of speech, body and conscious mind.

This is an area of conflict and difficulty for most women, not just those who suffer from vaginismus.

CAN WE INFLUENCE THE SUCCESS OF A TREATMENT?

There are no hard-and-fast rules which will guarantee a successful outcome, but factors (conscious and unconscious) may come into play that can either help or hinder the process. In reality it's only if a woman continues to express purely negative attitudes that success is unlikely, and the boundaries between hindering and helping are inevitably blurred. It is quite natural at times to have a combination of feelings which may both enhance and obstruct the therapeutic process.

Helping the Process

Any therapeutic experience can be greatly enhanced if the woman comes to it of her own accord, is highly motivated, and is prepared to work hard and endure a certain amount of pain. Naturally, such characteristics need to be matched by her therapist. The practitioners I spoke with all stress the importance of a trusting relationship between sufferer and therapist. Motivation is also cited as an important factor. One doctor adds how important it is that the woman's partner be loving and supportive. Generally, the likelihood of a favorable outcome is believed to be greater if the therapist

- has a capacity to understand our feelings.
- is skilled, sensitive, intuitive and patient.

If there is

- mutual trust
- willingness to confront our pain yet acknowledge our fears.
- motivation to change and grow.
- support from people.

And if we are

- willing to ask for support.
- able to express ourselves lovingly and enjoy intimacy.
- seeking help primarily to overcome vaginismus and not because of the desire for a baby.

- able to participate in the healing process and take responsibility when appropriate.
- open to success.

Hindering the Process

One doctor explained that success may be impeded if the woman does not feel safe enough to let go of her controls, reflecting an intimate partnership she may have.

A therapist working psychoanalytically says that the partner's unconscious conflicts can also interfere with progress:

> It could be that he's satisfied with the situation as it is, so that if the woman becomes more receptive and relaxed and things begin to shift in an internal way, it mightn't suit him.
> —Jill Curtis

Dr. Brown cites levels of fear that he cannot get underneath as impeding a successful outcome. He explains how the path of therapy can be obstructed by outside influences:

> One of the most difficult and unsuccessful attempts at treating vaginismus was where a priest was giving my client directly contrary advice at the same time.

For sex therapist Dr. Cole, it is a lack of knowledge about the true causes of vaginismus which may prevent him from intervening and may lead him to use the wrong approach for a particular woman.

The likelihood of a favorable outcome is accordingly believed to be less if the therapist

- lacks skills, sensitivity and ability to empathize.
- is unable to explore his or her countertransference toward the patient.
- is unaware of, or uninterested in, his or her own cultural stereotypes.

- is unaware of, or uninterested in, his or her unconscious conflicts surrounding sexuality.★

And if we

- remain ambivalent about confronting our problem.
- continue to resist change.
- only seek help because of external pressures.
- enter therapy because we feel humiliated that we are virgins rather than because we wish to enjoy intimacy.
- lack motivation.
- do not believe we can change or grow.
- feel negative toward ourselves, treatment, our partner and our therapist.
- continue to put up strong defenses.
- remain unable to recognize and make use of interpretations and insights.
- are unable to work with our fantasies, fail to distinguish them from reality and therefore cannot give them up.
- continue to see the relationship with our therapist as a struggle for power.
- continue to try and undermine the therapist's impact.
- continue to intellectualize, deny, withhold conscious thoughts and feelings and repress relevant material.
- remain passive, with no real engagement in the therapeutic relationship.
- continue to place the entire responsibility for change on the therapist.
- remain fearful of intimacy, dependence, trust and loss of control.
- remain closed to success.

★ See also the sections called "Creating Changes in Our Treatments" and "Openness About Risks of Therapy" (pages 229 and 230 of this chapter).

THE TREATMENTS: A PERSONAL VIEW

I include this very personal assessment of the treatments for three reasons. First, I wish to help women understand that there is no single right road to the resolution of vaginismus. However, I believe some women need to know this from a sufferer's firsthand experience, not just from a clinician's statistic.

Second, in being candid about the ways in which certain methods were inappropriate for me, I hope to enable women to consider the appropriateness of each treatment themselves rather than leaving their choice in the hands of an "expert." In making these observations about how and why a particular method failed for me, I hope to support the woman who may have difficulty in finding the right treatment and to show that it's OK if her first attempts do not succeed.

Third, much of women's pain, experience and history tends to go unnoticed in the world. Consequently, despite my wish not to offend the medical profession, I do not want to suppress the way in which some doctors treated me. I want other women to know that if similar things happened to them it was not necessarily their fault, but perhaps more to do with the doctor's unconscious conflicts combined with their own.

Understanding the Causes

Rather than inventing more cures and treatments for vaginismus, increasing concentration should be placed on the questions of *how* and *why* a woman has developed vaginismus in the first place. If we do not view vaginismus solely as a sexual problem, the obvious treatments will be ones which explore our psychology. While I tend to favor psychodynamic as opposed to strictly behavioral approaches, I am not in any way dismissing the value of the behavioral method. As we have seen, the practitioners I spoke with are all aware of the need to explore underlying conflicts rather than simply employing techniques to stretch women's vaginas and alter their behavior. What I cannot understand or support is the method which does not allow for the possibility of women's examining in their own time and their own way what the vaginismus is protecting them against. As Frances says:

> I feel quite irate about the sub-Masters-&-Johnson-cum-behavioral approach, which inevitably suggests that sensate focusing and the use of dilators and fingers will solve the problem in much the same automatic way that a pipe can be unblocked! I've never had any problem putting my fingers in my vagina, yet I still suffer from vaginismus.

The Move Away from Sexual Methods

My cautiousness about direct approaches may be unfounded in certain cases. For example, if a woman's difficulties occurred during later development but she has successfully negotiated the earlier phases or primary stages of her psychosexual development, behavioral therapy may well suit her. It may give her the green light to embark on sexuality. However, there may be drawbacks in this approach for the sufferer whose troubles date from a much earlier stage in her development. While she may well be able to function sexually after treatment, she may still be unable to feel loved and may continue to feel terrible deep inside.

If the pressure is removed to achieve penetration, a woman can more easily choose a method which explores underlying conflicts, since she will not feel dominated or pressured by the sexual aspects of the condition. It is not always appropriate or necessary to treat vaginismus with a sexual therapy, because sexual relationships cannot be separated from others. The issues of basic trust and allowing others into a woman's true self are pervasive in *every* relationship. It's possible to learn about a woman's sexuality simply by becoming aware of her interactions with others, without raising the subject of sex at all.

After much thought, research and discussion with sufferers and specialists, I remain unconvinced that one can simply bypass the deeper underlying conflicts of vaginismus and deal only with alleviating the symptom. As the section of this chapter called "Surgery" has shown, there may very well be a shift of symptoms, meaning that the spasm leaves the vagina but moves elsewhere. I am not alone in believing that vaginismus is developmental and that psychotherapy is the most appropriate form of treatment, this was also the conclusion of Dr. Friedman's *Virgin Wives*.

> It was only psychotherapy that enabled me to solve the problem . . . the dilators would have been useless without it.
>
> —Emma

However, as one psychoanalyst pointed out to me, some women don't take to therapy at first and may need to go through the disappointment and failure of the physical approaches. All of us have an unconscious resistance to looking inside ourselves, and this is reflected in our reluctance to enter the therapies which require us to do this.

Reappraising Treatments

Both past and contemporary publications appear to influence heavily the treatments for vaginismus. Prefeminist literature often refers to vaginismic women as "hostile" or "infantile"; this view came about mainly because the psychological measure of adulthood is genitally related, that is, whether or not a woman is able to allow penetration. If we remove the focus from the vagina it will not only produce a shift in the way vaginismic women are viewed, but also will save their partners from being judged in terms of masculinity or potency. Current approaches to sexual problems also appear to be too focused on the genitals. While it's true that many sexual problems manifest in one's vagina or penis, this may miss the true origins of the difficulty. Vaginismus has as much—or as little—to do with the vagina as anorexia nervosa has to do with the mouth.

Creating Changes in Our Treatments

As there may well be cultural, religious and ethnic influences which come into play in the makeup of our psychology, I feel it appropriate to set our psychology in the context of our social background when exploring vaginismus. I arrive at this conclusion since noticing and wondering why the incidence of vaginismus appears much higher among women in Ireland where there are strict religious taboos, than it is in England. Although the origins of vaginismus are diverse, Dr. Marian E. Dunn of the Center for Human Sexuality at the State University of New York Health Science Center points out that a restrictive and religious background may play a role in its onset:

> We see many Orthodox Jewish young women, and women from other religious backgrounds, who have been told that the first intercourse will be painful. I've noticed that in cultures that stress premarital virginity there is more of a tendency for young girls to be told frightening stories of how painful intercourse will be, perhaps to keep them from having sex before marriage. So in very religious families many young women have heard these stories. They also have had no premarital sexual experience because it's forbidden, and they've no sex education. The wedding night frequently is a very frightening time for the young woman, and often for the young man as well.

An awareness also needs to be developed of the ways in which class and race can affect a therapist's view of a sufferer. If a therapist remains blind to such issues, he may "psychologize" rather than explore them with the patient. The importance of examining the therapist's unconscious conflicts

about and feelings toward a patient is explained in Michael
Gorkin's *The Uses of Countertransference*. In the same way that
I suggested in "The Pelvic Examination" (page 203) that there
is a lack of information on the countertransference aspects of
treating vaginismus with a male gynecologist, Gorkin points
out that scant attention has been paid in the literature to
therapists' sexual feelings and fantasies about patients.[30] He
writes that while therapists continue to focus on the importance of countertransference in general, the specific domain
of sexualized countertransference needs to be further explored. Gorkin also pays particular attention to cultural and
ethnic influences by examining the relationship between Jewish Israeli therapists and their Arab patients. Interestingly,
though, many therapists do not consider that a man treating
a woman similarly needs to explore his culturally stereotyped
images of females!

By highlighting these aspects, I hope to stimulate a dialogue
about the treatments for vaginismus between every woman
and her doctor or therapist (as I suggested to gynecologists
in "The Pelvic Examination"). The methods by which we
currently treat vaginismus unconsciously reflect the way the
condition is seen; this is true for most problems and treatments. More support must be provided for practitioners to
explore, understand, and identify with sufferers and ultimately to bring compassion to the way a sufferer is seen and
treated.

Openness About the Risks of Therapy

Having explored the various treatments and therapies, it is
important to add that therapy is not a panacea for vaginismus,
and like everything worthwhile it carries a certain amount of
pain and risk. Dr. Peter Rutter in *Sex in the Forbidden Zone*
illustrates that abuses between male doctors or therapists and
female patients can and do occur, and he offers guidelines on
preventing them.[31] These issues may be especially relevant

to vaginismic women because of the intimate nature of the problem. I hope that increased awareness will generate more open discussions among the professionals who treat vaginismus.

A more extreme view warning against therapy was shared with me in a letter from Jeffrey Moussaieff Masson, an ex-psychoanalyst and author. He suggests to anybody who has "problems" that they find other people with the same problem, that they form self-help groups with no professionals, where no money changes hands, where there are no experts, and where the possibility of being further harmed is diminished. While Masson says he has many reservations about the religious dimensions of a group like Alcoholics Anonymous, he believes that something along those lines would be preferable to any kind of professional help.[32]

Because of my own experiences and those of other sufferers, I take a more moderate and optimistic view. I share the sentiments of Dr. M. Scott Peck, as stated in his afterword to *The Road Less Traveled*:

> Each person, therapist and patient is unique, and you must rely on your own unique intuitive judgment. Because there is some risk involved, I wish you luck. And because the act of entering psychotherapy with all that it involves is an act of courage, you have my admiration.[33]

I have compiled an appendix (beginning on page 269) listing various resources for women seeking treatment for vaginismus, both in the United States and in the United Kingdom. While I have been unable to provide a complete and definitive list, I have tried to cover as many regions as possible and all the different approaches to therapy that I have discussed. I hope that among the resources on the list you may find a starting place for your own treatment process.

Chapter 6

CAN VAGINISMUS
BE PREVENTED?

I don't see how we can prevent vaginismus because we're back to there being one cause . . . if you do this to your child it'll cause vaginismus or if you don't do this it won't.
—Jill Curtis, psychotherapist

I have wondered and wondered whether it is possible to prevent the occurrence of vaginismus. Since I have come to understand the origins of my vaginal spasm, I've asked myself whether this knowledge could be used to prevent its occurrence in a daughter of my own. While there is a growing emphasis on preventive medicine, it does not automatically follow that we can prevent psychological damage in a child as easily as we can lessen the dangers of physical harm by keeping poisons out of reach and teaching our children how to cross the street safely. Life is a continuum from birth to death, and no matter how important certain events are, it is never *one* incident that causes anything. People who experience trauma in early life can often lead very happy existences if positive influences follow to counteract the negative ones. Therefore, it should not be assumed that our insensitivity or natural errors in raising our children will definitely cause vaginismus, or any emotional problem. Other factors should always be considered, such as the inherent emotional makeup of children and their own particular needs.

Realistically, there is little anyone can do to prevent the

onset of vaginismus. Thinking back to Chapter Three, there is probably a limit to how much good mothering can prevent or alter the fantasies a baby has . . . fantasies which may be influential in the development of vaginismus. This is because they develop before an infant is able to make rational judgments about external events or her parents' behavior toward her. While it's true that the mother plays a vital role in providing a secure environment in which a baby's psychological self can develop in a healthy way, she is in no way responsible for the development of vaginismus, since it is never caused by her knowingly "doing" something to her baby. As Swedish therapist Marianne Granö explains:

> Parents can't prevent vaginismus because most try consciously to be good parents. They are all the time carrying their own lives, their own mothers and fathers with them.

To say that vaginismus cannot be prevented may seem pessimistic, but if we look at prevention within a much wider framework, possibilities open up. Rather than trying to prevent an unconscious interaction between infant and parent, we need to look at it in terms of understanding how and why sexual and emotional problems like vaginismus may arise as a result of such an interaction.

THE FAMILY'S ROLE

The growing general awareness and openness about the causes and existence of vaginismus may help to raise the consciousness of parents, alerting them to the importance of sensitivity in their interactions with their children. Even quite simple insights into a child's psychological life can help us to understand how crucial early emotional experiences are in shaping our futures.

Most parents want to do the best for their children. Unfortunately, there are so many ways of harming a child, and it can be done unintentionally and unconsciously. It's often easier for us, through fear, ignorance and social conditioning, to hold our children back than it is to help them reach their full potential. Instead of blaming others, it might be more positive to accept the difficulties in being a parent and acknowledge that most mistakes can be repaired with love and understanding, as well as an acceptance of our responsibilities. The suggestions in this chapter are not intended as a guide to good parenting, since none of them, either on their own or in combination, can definitely prevent the occurrence of vaginismus. However, increased consciousness and thought might lessen the possibility. There is no such thing as a perfect parent, and strange as it may seem, it is possible to be too good a parent. Donald Winnicott points out that problems can arise when mothers are so experienced at reading their children's needs that they anticipate them all and thus unwittingly rob their children of the experience of disappointment and of gaining control for themselves.[1] We need somehow to maintain that delicate balance between wanting to satisfy our children totally and realizing that this is neither realistically possible nor healthy.

A CHILD'S VIEW OF THE ADULT

Perhaps more useful than reading child-rearing manuals is a parent's developing the ability to "become" the child, to feel a child's feelings and to see things from her perspective. If we understand that a girl feels ambivalent toward her mother because her mother is the source of both her happiness and her pain, we can more easily allow that child to express negative and hateful feelings as well as loving ones.

We need to recognize and become more sensitive to a child's awareness of adult relationships and sexuality. Psychoanalysis confirms that the "primal scene" may all too easily be misinterpreted, leading to erroneous assumptions which arise out of intense unconscious feelings of exclusion. If a child's exposure to the primal scene is not handled thoughtfully, she may be left feeling unable to compete with her mother, which can instill a sense of terror should she try to trespass on her mother's sexual territory by competing for her father's love.

However hard it may be to accept, we need to acknowledge that even very small children may have unconscious incestuous feelings and fantasies about their parents. Similarly, parents may also experience unconscious erotic feelings for their children. By acknowledging to ourselves that this is a natural process, we can allow a child to mature without undue guilt or anxiety. However, this does not give license to parents to overtly question children about such feelings, or to act on any desires they might have themselves. The process goes on inside a child's unconscious and should be left there to work itself out quietly, free from inappropriate intrusion.

Another important aspect of the parent-child relationship is the boundary which must exist between them. For the adult this involves acting within a responsible framework, not imposing sexual or emotional demands on our children or expecting them to meet our needs. For the child it's simply the reassurance of knowing that the relationship with her parents is clearly defined, relieving her of any anxieties she might have about crossing boundaries. She is then able to happily engage in childhood rather than become prematurely involved in or confused by the demands of adults.

Psychologist Dr. Paul Brown highlights the importance of this aspect:

> The family's role is knowing how to be both private and relaxed about sex, and how to have boundaries around important issues like one's sexual development.

SELF-IMAGE, SELF-LOVE AND SELF-WORTH

We must recognize that the origins of poor self-esteem, lack of self-worth and self-love, and a negative self-image can often be traced to unsupportive, unpraising and dismissive attitudes toward a child from its parents. Early feelings of ugliness, unimportance and self-loathing may later reemerge, making it impossible, for example, for a woman to open up and share with others her true self, including her vaginismus.

Since early detection of children's problems is always preferable to allowing them to continue unnoticed beyond adolescence, we need to be acutely aware of any anxieties our children are consistently communicating.

Positive attitudes communicated to children about sex and their bodies can go far to promote healthy growth without undue fear of sex.

> If a girl is deprived of understanding and touching her vagina, it may build up into a psychological barrier that she mustn't do it.
>
> —Barbara Lamb, nurse-psychosexual counselor

If parents feel comfortable and at ease with their own sexuality, they are more likely to transmit positive messages to their children about sex.

A 1987 survey in a women's magazine revealed that little girls whose fathers are accessible rather than distant are more likely to be orgasmic and enjoy their sexuality.[2] This demonstrates that "being there" for one's child is important not only for her psychological welfare but also for her sexual development.

AN INFANT'S NEED TO FEEL LOVED AND SECURE

We don't live in an ideal world, but whenever possible we should avoid leaving a baby unattended for unreasonably long periods to cry alone. This may instill a sense of isolation, unhappiness, loneliness and insecurity, leading her to expect that nobody will ever come to relieve her of her misery, which may then result in her subsequently mistrusting and hating the entire world, seeing it as hostile, unsafe and cruelly withholding.

Women who encourage independence in their children because they feel relatively secure and fulfilled generally fare better as mothers than those who are emotionally troubled or immature. Unresolved conflicts in a woman's personality, combined with social factors, may result in her needing her baby to boost her ego, making it difficult for a child to separate psychologically from her mother. This inability to separate and ultimately own one's self—including one's vagina—is particularly noticeable in women who go on to develop vaginismus.

MOTHER NOT SEEN AS THE EXPERT

While it's commonly recognized that the mother is essential to her infant, paradoxically she is not considered the expert. We are encouraged to draw on outside expertise, consulting books and professionals. It's hardly surprising that women come to feel insecure about whether their responses to their babies are the "right" ones. Perhaps we need to be encouraged more to trust our own feelings.

> On the one hand motherhood is deified . . . and on the other hand it is undermined.
>
> —Susie Orbach, psychotherapist

Out of insecurity and a desire to be model parents, many of us rely on rigid feeding schedules rather than spontaneous and intuitive responses to baby's physical and emotional needs. This may lead to a child's not feeling special or feeling that she does not have unique qualities which need attending to in a unique way. If we are not encouraged to see children as individuals, we may forget they are "real" and be clumsy and unintentionally brutal in our handling of them. This can lead a child to assume that the world is clumsy and not to be trusted. It can take a long time to renounce such a belief and come to trust others.

While parents-to-be are inundated with books and instructions on how to breathe through the contractions of labor and how to feed and change the baby, very little emphasis is placed on the emotional lives of parent and child. Many adults may have no psychological sense of what goes on for the baby throughout her emotional development; the education of parents, teachers, nursery workers and other caretakers needs to be reappraised. Without appropriate education, the language of psychology may remain a jargon of the elite. To help remedy this, prenatal classes need to include information not just about diaper-changing but also about the emotional aspects of child-rearing:

> A parent needs to have a sense of her own emotional life as an adult in order to be receptive to the potential emotional life of her infant.
>
> —Susie Orbach

BECOMING A PARENT RE-EVOKES THE BABY IN US

In the same way that a therapist cannot be taught how to feel and be intuitive, parents cannot learn awareness and sensitivity simply from psychoanalytic "lessons." Instead, we need to be helped to understand that it is not only what we do to our children, but how we feel when we do it that matters. For example, many of us may be unaware just how sensitive a baby is to the emotional attitudes of her caregivers. For this reason, it's far better to have a relaxed, happy mother feeding to a schedule than an anxious and resentful one who breast-feeds on demand.

When problems arise in the way a parent relates intimately to her infant, they usually spring from unconscious emotional conflicts which stem from the mother's own childhood. When a woman becomes a mother, powerful emotions are re-evoked which have a great deal in common with feelings stirred up in her by her parents and siblings when she herself was a child. The way she feels toward her baby is often distorted by unconscious early conflicts she reexperiences, leading her perhaps to respond in inappropriate ways. However, the difficulty is not in this recurrence of feelings, which all of us experience as parents, but rather in a mother's or father's inability to understand, recognize, tolerate and control the feelings.[3] Much guilt and confusion could be alleviated if we were helped to recognize that a needy, possibly deprived baby inside us is always re-created when we have a child.

HEALING INEQUALITIES AMONG MOTHER, FATHER AND BABY

When discussing the issue of prevention, Susie Orbach explained that she sees vaginismus as being no different from other psychological symptoms. In other words, it is really about difficulties in relating intimately, and the terror and desire that produces. Part of any effort at prevention would be to change the cultural atmosphere around the whole issue of intimacy:

> We are illiterate when it comes to intimate relationships, so we need to change the illiteracy of emotional contact rather than simply introduce procedures to "deal with" or "prevent" vaginismus.

It follows that issues surrounding the way we relate intimately need to be understood and explored. Since the all-important figure at the start of life is usually the mother, perhaps it's here we can effect change. Are there ways to help limit the conditions which give rise to vaginismus?

The authors of the book *What Do Women Want?* suggest that changing the position of women in society will help change the psychological makeup of women.[4] This requires involving men equally in child-rearing to alter men's psychology. As nurturers, men will experience the same feelings of inadequacy, anxiety and vulnerability that women currently experience.

The results of this might be:

- Dependence will no longer be seen to signify weakness.
- Our needs for contact, care, intimacy and love will be accepted as natural.
- Two parents of different genders can help a baby tolerate painful experiences and so make her feel she can survive them, that they are not dangerous, overwhelming or ugly.
- All badness or neurosis and distrust will no longer be seen as deriving from disappointment with mothers or other women (the root of misogyny in male psychology?) because both good and bad experiences will be associated with both parents.

SOCIETY'S ROLE

What can we as a society collectively do to reduce the occurrence and the stigma of vaginismus?

A HEALTHY SEXUAL CLIMATE

We need to encourage a climate in which sexuality and intimacy are expressed, not just openly, but without derision, shame, or embarrassment, and with respect for its specialness and sacredness. Ways in which such a climate might be created are:

- Recognition that sex needs to be seen within a more holistic framework. This means integrating our sexuality with the other aspects of ourselves, rather than separating it. Separation of sex removes it from the whole persons we are, leading to its compartmentalization, to our putting sex in one box and love in another. Such divisions reinforce women being seen as property and sex as a commodity, or as a male weapon used to dominate and oppress women.

• Acknowledgment that sex is the deepest expression of human creativity and communication, and consequently carries with it emotions of great depth and complexity. Unresolved pain related to intimacy can ultimately lead to its abuse and derision, or become a reason for pornography, prostitution, incest, promiscuity and celibacy.

• No longer seeing penile penetration as "it" or as the definitive proof of a loving relationship. In the most intimate and private aspect of a couple's life, they can feel pressured to conform and compete with norms of sex, losing sight of the fact that sexuality is an important aspect of self-expression. Instead, the union between a man and a woman should be judged more by the quality of their mutual love and devotion than by their ability to achieve penetration. This erroneous measure of love and commitment cruelly dismisses all vaginismic marriages as unconsummated and therefore invalid, even those lasting well beyond twenty years.

• Recognition that sexual problems are common, not rare, and that very few people may actually have a completely healthy attitude toward sex, sexuality and their bodies.

• Emphasizing the powerful healing forces that exist in communication and awareness of and respect for sexuality: Increased communication about vaginismus is healing, since it can lead to the uncovering of other unspoken sexual issues. So, too, is increased awareness, since this can lead to the removal of stigma and taboo surrounding sexual problems. Increased respect for sexuality will also actively discourage our propensity to ridicule, making it inappropriate to mock people who have sexual problems.

· Recognition of the resistance we all have to being truly open in talking about sex.

· Recognizing that continually suppressing the truth about painful issues such as vaginismus ultimately makes it more difficult for women to come forward and equally difficult for vaginismus to be recognized and understood.

· Within the past few years, the sexual climate has been radically altered by the advent of AIDS. Couples (straight and gay) are now encouraged, at least at the start of a relationship, to practice safe sex. Not only a safety measure (which can also feel like a hindrance), safe sex has also expanded people's awareness that there are other erotic pleasures besides penetration. It is very important for vaginismic couples to feel that making love without intercourse is still making love.

LEARNING ABOUT SEXUAL LOVE
FROM THE ANCIENT PAST

There was a time (as in ancient China) when women played prominent roles in forming the philosophy of a society; and when their position has been equal to that of men, sexual practices have reflected that equality. However, when society changes from matriarchy to patriarchy, the balance in the sexual act shifts radically. As our role degenerates into a subordinate one, so does the focus on our sexual satisfaction. The notion that psychological health is connected to one's ability to relate intimately is not new; Taoist masters predate Freud by many thousands of years. *Tao* is the Chinese word for "path" or "way" and represents the Chinese system of religion and philosophy which looks at life and its relation to eternal truth. Current Western attitudes toward sex, including its derision and pornography, are distinctly opposed to Oriental teachings. The Tao art of loving has three basic principles, which were put forward and accepted in the West mainly through the work of Masters & Johnson and the women's liberation movement[5]:

- recognizing that female satisfaction is crucial
- understanding that ejaculation can and should be regulated and delayed
- understanding that male orgasm and ejaculation are not one and the same

At one time or another many men may suffer from impotence. Unlike Westerners, the ancient Chinese never saw this as an important problem. Here, the words "impotent" and "frigid" are overused, misused and pejorative. The Taoists believe a man can still enter a woman by the "soft entry" method, penetrating without an erection and using his fingers to guide him. Once inside, there is a good chance he can become erect. Soft entry shatters two myths about male sexuality: that a man cannot enter a woman unless he has achieved an erection, and that the erection must be very strong in order to penetrate.

Soft entry may also remove the pressure from anyone who is experiencing difficulty in achieving penetration.

Many practitioners stress that sufferers from vaginismus should be encouraged to seek help early so that they do not carry the condition and the shameful feelings that accompany it around for years. If the emphasis was removed from penetration and "impotence," it would help erase the stigma of vaginismus, enabling us to seek help without shame.

While openness about sex is important, quality may be more critical than quantity. The apparent freedom of the

media to discuss intimate issues may sometimes give us a
false sense of openness:

> What's discussed about sexuality doesn't go far enough, so
> it's assumed people have trivial problems. This means dis-
> cussions about sex need to be about trying to understand the
> experience from the sufferer's point of view.
>
> —Susie Orbach

SEX EDUCATION FOR CHILDREN AND ADULTS

A healthy and wholesome attitude toward sex should be encouraged early, starting with the education of young children.
Because pornography is a source of misinformation, we need
to recognize that reeducation may be necessary for us all. As
well as being informed about sex, children need to hear not
only that it is good and welcome, but also that it involves
some decision-making.

> We need to highlight both the pleasure of sex and the re-
> sponsibility it carries.
>
> —Dr. Paul Brown

JOINT SUPPORT FROM FAMILY AND SOCIETY

A healthier sexual climate would not just benefit children but
would also encourage adults to break taboos about conditions
such as vaginismus and not perpetuate its concealment or the
myth that it is rare. Without the shame, secrecy and fear of
ridicule, a sufferer would feel less traumatized and unnatural.
If vaginismus became more widely acknowledged and understood, women would not have to suffer in silence but would
be able to seek support, not only from professionals, but also
from much-needed family and friends. The enormous pressures that are sometimes insensitively placed on a woman
who has not yet made her mother a grandmother may often
increase her pain and despair:

Women don't normally go to their families and say they have vaginismus, and it's sad because spasm is not deliberate . . . parents need to understand their daughter is a normal person.

—Barbara Lamb

SPEAKING OUT AGAINST VIOLENCE AND SEXUAL ABUSE

Evidence exists to support the belief that vaginismus may develop after childhood sexual abuse or rape. It follows that the safer the environment, the less incidence there will be of vaginismus. Responsibility falls on all of us to both help the abused and treat the offender, since sexual violence is often committed by people who were themselves abused:

I go into prisons and talk about vaginismus with rapists. I explain that their crime isn't something written on a page . . . what they've actually given a woman is an inability to make love. I tell them how when I was raped I had this "block" and couldn't be penetrated, and one of the rapists identified with this . . . something in him seemed to click.

—Jan

It may also be that a woman who is being physically abused by her partner is not able to tell him she suffers from vaginismus. It is therefore very important that men understand exactly what vaginismus is, further helping to end the shame and secrecy that currently exist.

THE DOCTOR'S ROLE

Because the majority of women who suffer from vaginismus will receive treatment from a member of the medical profession, the importance of the doctor's role in resolving vaginismus should not be underestimated.

CREATING A POSITIVE ATTITUDE
TOWARD SEX AND CHILDBIRTH

More open attitudes toward sex would undoubtedly benefit doctors as well as the rest of us, since they are exposed to the same sexual influences in society as everyone else. Less repressed, less judgmental attitudes would create an opening for doctors to explore, understand and accept their own anxieties about intimacy. This might then encourage a less fearful atmosphere when treating vaginismus.

Many midwives and obstetricians stress the importance of an enjoyable, natural birth experience for mothers and babies, believing that childbirth should be less medicalized, giving more power, choice and emotional support to the woman. As we learned in Chapter Three, the mother-daughter relationship is a crucial one in the developing psychology of an infant. Postnatal studies confirm that a less uncomfortable and less frightening labor can increase a mother's self-esteem, enabling her to feel more secure and confident in her new motherhood. Such positive feelings are likely to be transmitted to an infant daughter, helping to give the baby a sense of her body's future power and creativity, rather than a sense of fear, passivity and negativity.

PUTTING SEX ON THE CURRICULUM
FOR MEDICAL STUDENTS

The medical community also has a professional responsibility to ensure that future generations of doctors are well informed about vaginismus. One way is to introduce human sexuality programs as an *essential* part of the curriculum in medical schools.

For example, students could be taught how to diagnose vaginismus early, rather than leaving it to be discovered in a prenatal exam or maternity ward, or in older women when the resultant treatment may be more difficult and protracted.

The more medical students are supported in trying to understand themselves, the more likely they are to be able to identify and work with their future patients' sexual problems. If a doctor's training leaves him ill prepared to recognize vaginismus, he may mistakenly diagnose an intact hymen or simply give treatment for a nonexistent infection. Even worse, he may dismiss the woman's anguish with the reassurance that "it will fix itself in the end." As I have already explained, one well-intentioned doctor told me to "go away and get drunk" before attempting intercourse. The Association of American Medical Colleges confirms that 23 medical schools list "Human Sexuality" *as a required course*; 79 offer "Human Sexuality" as an elective course; and 110 indicate they teach "Human Sexuality" as part of a required course.

PSYCHOSEXUAL TRAINING FOR PRIMARY CARE PHYSICIANS

As discussed in the previous chapter, the primary care setting may be the most appropriate in which to treat vaginismus. It takes tremendous courage for many women with vaginismus to seek help, and if a woman's first contact is likely to be the family physician it would be so much better if he or she was psychosexually trained.

The American Medical Association confirms that, as in the United Kingdom, there is no mandatory postgraduate training in the United States for primary care physicians in treating vaginismus. Such training may be given to doctors in an OB/GYN residency, who will encounter vaginismus in their daily work. In the case of the primary care physician, while he or she is legally required to take a certain amount of training through continuing education programs, the choice of program is left to the doctor.

The notion that sufferers from vaginismus are so difficult to treat that it requires a specialist with particular training may reinforce the idea that we are somehow more tricky and demanding than other patients. We are not. It has also been pointed out that for a primary care physician to respond with "Ah, yes . . . I know an excellent expert for you" (even if he or she does) may merely increase our sense of abnormality.[6]

Since training in the treatment of vaginismus is not yet mandatory, all that may be required of many primary care physicians to treat this condition is increased awareness and empathy, patience and persistence.

ENCOURAGING SENSITIVITY AMONG MEDICAL PRACTITIONERS

As we know, in some instances the woman's general practitioner may not be her first contact. It is therefore important that greater focus be placed on sensitivity for *all* doctors. Vaginismus might make a doctor feel powerless because it prevents him from being able to examine a woman, but he could be helped to understand that she is not consciously resisting examination. While the woman's fears and feelings about being examined may seem totally irrational to the doctor, he should nevertheless accept that for her they are real and need to be acknowledged.

Sadly, some doctors who encounter vaginismus (perhaps due to their own suppressed sexual conflicts, or inadequate training) unconsciously project their frustration and exasperation onto women who suffer from vaginismus. My experiences match those of others whose vaginismus was received by some doctors with impatience and intolerance instead of empathy and understanding. This may often make the therapeutic relationship unnecessarily painful.

> The doctors get cross because it makes them feel they're not very good. They are defeated by women who have vaginismus and often can't cope with their anger.
> —Dr. Katharine Draper, member,
> Institute of Psychosexual Medicine

Although both may be involved in treating vaginismus, doctors and psychotherapists come from very different backgrounds. It is the nature of psychotherapy that the therapist explores and understands his own conflicts regarding a condition, whereas doctors tend to remain detached and are not encouraged to examine their own feelings. Because of the unconscious conflicts induced in the doctor when confronted with anorexia or vaginismus (conditions in which a woman can be seen to be making some kind of protest) the sufferer is often silenced by the physician, either by his insistence on treating her symptoms inappropriately or by shouting at her in frustration. To add to this, it is a two-way phenomenon, in that the woman is also silenced by her own shame.

> Practitioners need to try and put themselves into the woman's skin and feel the terror, despair, shame and humiliation that a symptom induces. Doctors often aren't very good at doing this, they aren't trained to deal with the distress they encounter. As a result they may distance themselves from the patient.
>
> —Susie Orbach

We all need to be particularly careful to avoid making an assumption that all women have had sexual intercourse. This is particularly true of doctors working in VD clinics. The automatic assumption that a married or older woman is not a virgin might lead to vaginal examinations being carried out in a less gentle and sensitive manner. As explained, traumatic internals may compound vaginismus even further.

THE DOCTOR–NURSE TEAM

In "Louise's Treatment" in Chapter Five we saw that nurses play a valuable role in treating vaginismus. In Sweden, for example, family planning is taken care of by midwives, so many are naturally involved in treating vaginismus. Marianne Granö explains the advantages of this:

In our clinic, as with many other family planning clinics in Sweden, we mostly work with midwives. Doctors and midwives working closely with sexual counselors have more experience and a more personal way of handling a difficult vaginal examination.

The nature of vaginismus makes it a very sensitive and delicate issue. It may, therefore, respond more positively to the more equal relationship that generally exists between patient and nurse. Physicians, whatever their gender, are often perceived as all-knowing and all-powerful, which may create an imbalance and a distance between them and their patients. It is important for a woman to feel that she is on the same level as her practitioner; when she does, she experiences her treatment as more under her control. A nursing background can enhance a sense of equality between practitioner and client:

> Our approach toward treating vaginismus is holistic. We tend to use our perceptions more and go slowly; we take a detailed history and then work jointly with a therapist.
> —Mimi Clark Secor, registered nurse-practitioner

Because of the obvious emotional benefits outlined here, coupled with the financial advantages (less intervention, more cost-effective), training for nurses in the treatment of vaginismus needs to be encouraged and advanced.

Awareness, sensitivity and collaboration are the ways forward in improving the treatment of vaginismus. Marianne Granö, for example, believes that psychotherapists and gynecologists are too far apart:

> We need to work more closely with the gynecologists. We are both very much needed in treating sexual problems, but the ideal combination is to work together in the beginning.

NEW AGE MEDICINE:
THE ARRIVAL OF HOLISTIC GYNECOLOGY?

Rina Nissim's approach to treating vaginismus might well represent the beginning of holistic gynecology—that is, a closer collaboration between therapy and gynecology such as Marianne Granö hopes for:

> First what is really to be "treated"? The vagina, the sexuality or the compulsory penetration? What is vaginismus if not part of oneself which does not want intercourse and a conflict with the will, and the will of one's partner?
> —Rina Nissim, feminist health worker, Geneva

Nissim explains that sexuality comes not out of politics but rather from a field of power relationships, and unless one considers vaginismus in this context any treatment is not holistic. She stresses that focusing on facilitating penile penetration is too local or mechanical, adding:

> It is essentially a discussion concerning sexuality in individual consultation which is needed to understand a woman's conflicting interests. I often suggest that she give up trying to have intercourse for six months in order to discover something else, to "degenitalize" sexuality, and try to pass over her block by reconsidering her whole sexuality instead of trying to force it locally. This is what we mean by holistic gynecology.

Things are changing in the medical world, with many more physicians favoring the "whole person" (holistic) approach to medicine, rather than simply viewing symptoms in isolation. Members of the American Holistic Medical Association and the British Holistic Medical Association★ approach the experience of disorder from the human perspective.

Homeopath Dr. Kenneth Metson believes his branch of medicine can and should play a much larger role in the treat-

★ For details, see Appendix, page 274.

ment of vaginismus. He explained that many general practitioners refer patients to him if they are not responding to conventional medication:

> Alternative medicine should definitely be given consideration if a woman with vaginismus hasn't had success with other treatments.

Because vaginismus should ideally be seen as a symptom reflecting a woman's whole being, it is hoped that all practitioners (medical and nonmedical) will approach the treatment of vaginismus within a holistic framework and with minimum physical intervention. This kind of approach would give us back our power to:

- take responsibility for our health
- question
- be seen as the experts on our own bodies
- be autonomous and able to fulfill our creative potential

ACCEPTING REALITY

No matter how sensitive and aware we all may try to be, and no matter how skilled and kind medical professionals are, we must realistically accept that although we may try to plan for a perfect future, reality often fails to meet our utopian expectations. Part of human experience is that we inevitably fail in certain areas; we may lack empathy for others or inadvertently hurt those we love. We need to be humble in recognizing our confusion and admitting, "Yes—maybe there are better ways of dealing with problems which we don't yet know about," and "Yes—we have still so much to learn."

If we can maintain a goal to be as loving, aware and sensitive as possible, and be able to acknowledge it when we fall short, surely we can make a valuable contribution to increased understanding of, and ultimately prevention of, vaginismus, as well as a host of other problems.

Chapter 7

FREE! TO LET
IN LOVE AND TRUST

The courageous journey that a woman takes in confronting, understanding and resolving vaginismus may often involve a mixture of confusion, hate, despair, pain, fear, relief and love. Similarly, the journey through this book may have re-evoked some of these emotions. In this final chapter I, along with others, describe what resolution means for us. For some it is the arrival at a sense of belonging to themselves; for others, the freedom to express themselves sexually. In fairy tales, people always live happily ever after, but in reality I prefer to see the resolution of a problem more in terms of a strengthening process than as an end in itself. Knowing that there may always be obstacles to overcome, and knowing, too, that we are able to resolve them, are far more empowering than believing happiness only exists when there are no problems.

RESOLUTION AS A CONTINUING PROCESS

A chapter on resolution would not be complete without an acknowledgment of the women who, for a variety of reasons, have been unable to resolve their vaginismus. The inclusion of sufferers who have not yet reached resolution is a way of saying that they, too, can be part of transformation and success. It may be that the experiences shared in this book will lead them to seek help and support. In time I hope it will become easier for us to come forward and talk about our pain, and for others to respond to vaginismus more imaginatively and sensitively:

> So here I am . . . middle-aged . . . having an awful menopause, longing for lots of sex but unable to do anything about it.

> My husband has stuck by me, and we are happy in our own way. Everyone has something to contend with, and this is our cross.

> I felt so humiliated when I last sought help that I will never seek it again. I try to forget about it . . . it's difficult, but you get used to it as time goes on.

> Actually, I haven't entirely given up hope . . . maybe there's a cure somewhere . . . I'd like to know of alternatives . . . What's worked for other people?

> I'm not bitter, just very sad at what we've had to miss all our married lives.

> I still haven't given up. Always is the hope that something will work . . . someone can hypnotize me out of my fear . . . or there'll be a magic pill . . . I keep hoping for a miracle.

> I've given up this year . . . hope at last has gone . . . I'll never be better and will have to face it.

I would like to say to these women, and to any one who has yet to receive appropriate help: don't ever give up . . . even if you haven't yet found the right help, persevere. You have a right to be free, to be your own person, and to have control over your own body.

RESOLUTION OF THE SPASM

For doctors and therapists, transformation may be more easily defined. Most, for example, remark how different women look after they no longer suffer from vaginismus:

She walks in with a smile on her face and a pride in herself because she knows she's the only person who's actually made this happen.

—Dr. Robina Thexton, Member,
Institute of Psychosexual Medicine

Nurse-therapist Barbara Lamb says she can tell the moment a woman walks into the clinic that she has resolved her vaginismus:

The relief on her face is quite wonderful.

Dr. Paul Brown describes transformation in romantic terms, likening a woman's resolution to her "falling in love all over again."

Therapist Dr. Martin Cole said that normally he does not talk about "cure" when treating sexual problems, but adds:

Vaginismus is one of the few conditions where there is a qualitative change.

However, not all therapists see resolution in such clearly defined terms:

It's a process more than a transformation, and the progress can go up and down.

—Marianne Granö, sexual psychotherapist, Sweden

The actual spotlight on the vaginismus goes, and shifts from the vagina to the whole of the personality where the woman moves into a more in–depth way of looking at herself and her inner world.

—Jill Curtis, psychotherapist

SO WHAT IS RESOLUTION?

I accept that the ways in which I see resolution may not be acknowledged on a general level or by practitioners who may be looking more for the disappearance of spasm. However, my vaginismus became less of a total block as I noticed other areas in my life opening up. For me, transformation did not necessarily take place at the point when I no longer suffered from vaginismus, but rather when I saw healing my condition as a process and less of an unattainable goal. The key to resolution is in this process itself—that is, understanding the reasons for vaginismus and the ways in which we develop it. This shift of emphasis is more likely to take place if:

- vaginismus is relocated to the areas of love, mutual dependence, intimacy and trust as opposed to a woman's sexuality.

- the focus on penetration is removed to allow us to explore the deeper underlying causes. Continually seeing vaginismus as a sexual rather than an emotional problem not only pressures us into seeking therapies which may be inappropriate or ignore the unconscious, but also perpetuates the labeling of a woman and her partner.

- vaginismus is not deemed to be resolved when the symptom is alleviated, but rather when body and mind are in harmony.

Removing the focus from sex to the emotions may also create space to discuss wider issues surrounding vaginismus, related to other emotional blocks. For example, one friend said that learning about vaginismus has made her wonder just how many women suffer from psychological vaginismus— that is, a condition in which a woman can allow her lover to penetrate her vagina but not her heart, soul or mind.

GOALS BECOMING BLOCKS

My idealization of the act of penetration took on such enormous proportions that I became unable to let go and let growth, change and love inside. In effect, my goal became part of my unconscious closedness. If resolution is judged to occur only when we no longer have the spasm, the periods when we feel closed, depressed or have slight difficulty with lovemaking might seem enormous setbacks. If a therapy is too goal-oriented, it may make us feel desperately that unless we reach *the* cause we will not achieve resolution. As we have seen, there is never just one cause of vaginismus; therefore, such narrow goals may perpetuate our hopelessness. A treatment which seeks to remove the focus from the vagina can enable us to refrain from constantly measuring success in terms of penetration or self-examination. Whenever I attempted to examine myself forcefully, my analyst interpreted it as an attack on both myself and the process of therapy. I was also helped to recognize that constantly focusing on my inability to have sex somehow kept my vaginismus in place.

Goals are not unimportant. The point is that they should not become blocks to resolving vaginismus. It may be more helpful if goals are set which can be achieved today rather than tomorrow. For example, a constant aim of mine was to have a baby. When I understood that this longing also represented my need to give and receive loving feelings, I made it my goal to be able to feel and give love in the present. The goal of having a baby no longer seemed such a huge and unattainable achievement at a time when penetration was not yet possible.

Redefining Vaginismus

It can be powerfully healing to change the dialogue we engage in about our problems. Though this may seem too subtle a change to be effective, I noticed that altering the way I spoke about vaginismus produced a shift in the way I felt. For example, when I first began writing I planned to call this book *Women Who Can't Make Love*. Then, as I started to feel free from the spasm on levels other than the vaginal, I saw that in continuing to say "I can't make love" I was actually having the same conversation about vaginismus that I despised others for having (that is, defining sexual ability purely in terms of penetration). It seemed hypocritical to expect others to view vaginismus in a more enlightened way if I was not prepared to do it myself, so I abandoned the use of judgmental language. I was then able to acknowledge that although I could not engage in penetration I was certainly able to be loving. Consequently, changing my way of speaking led me to change the title of this book.

Changing our attitude can also extend to the way we define vaginismus in relation to our selves.[1] I felt deeply ashamed of my condition and discovered that I was not alone in these feelings. We only have to think of Valerie's statement that she would have to emigrate if anyone found out she has vaginismus. If I am defined by myself and others solely as someone with vaginismus, and this has negative connotations, it is hard for me not to see this part of myself as ugly, repulsive and overwhelming. We need to be helped to move beyond this limited definition and begin to see that vaginismus has nothing to do with our beauty, creativity, or ability to care and love, and to see that we possess other qualities. Eventually, vaginismus will not automatically trigger responses of repulsion or shame but instead may be seen as just one part of the whole of a woman, not the single defining characteristic.[2] I am more than my vaginismus.

True, the spasm represents the angry, hurt, unloved parts of myself, but it is not the total Linda. No woman should ever feel she has to emotionally emigrate for shame of who she is. She is a whole person, not just the vaginismus.

SHARING AS PART OF THE SOLUTION

Resolution of vaginismus may take very different forms. For me, part of it has been in writing this book, and part of it has been in the sharing of myself with others. As time passed and my ego grew stronger, it became less of an ordeal to tell each person about my vaginismus. My greatest discovery was the transformation this produced in my relationships with others and theirs with me. Perhaps because I have spent so long struggling with my sexuality and the anguish that vaginismus has brought to my life, I feel a particular sensitivity toward other people's pain. Sometimes this may take the form of awareness that something painful is going on for a person without my knowing exactly what the problem is. For example, one friend tearfully confided that she and her partner had not been able to make love for more than two years. After her disclosure she apologized, saying she didn't know why she'd told me but instinctively knew I'd understand. I then told her about my vaginismus. For so long the isolation and secrecy of my condition had made me feel I was the only woman who had problematic sex or no sex. It helped me to see that other women's sexuality may also be a painful issue and that it is not shameful to have a sexual problem. Only when there is less suppression will we be able to speak honestly about our difficulties.

Other Women Feel Envious and Excluded, Too

The woman who succeeds in overcoming vaginismus may feel affirmation of her womanhood as well as a sense of inclusion in areas from which she had previously felt excluded. However, in talking about mutual experiences, some of my friends admitted having similar feelings of exclusion and envy regarding sex, couples and pregnancy. A recently divorced friend admitted that she could not bear being in the presence of couples or even hearing about weddings; another revealed that the announcement of a friend's pregnancy had made her feel envious and excluded. Neither of these women suffer from vaginismus, yet both had experienced emotions similar to mine. This was a revelation to me. For as long as I could remember I had harbored guilt and remorse because of my feelings about the very same issues.

I realized that feelings of envy and exclusion are not unique to me, nor are they some kind of sinister pathology belonging only to a woman with vaginismus. They are part of universal human experience. Through analysis I learned that the same emotionally charged events (pregnancy, exclusivity of couples in relationships) may trigger primitive feelings in women who do not have vaginismus, and that such emotions originate in infancy.

Pride, Relief and Freedom

With the relief from longstanding feelings of shame and secrecy comes freedom to decide whether or not to become a mother. The rewards may be almost as great for the doctor as for the woman who has at last been able to reach this step:

Women thank me and send me cards announcing the births of their babies.

—Dr. Robina Thexton

However, it isn't just the ability to become a mother which marks happiness and freedom. For some, motherhood is not a desire, and for others it is sadly not possible. The most important factor is being able to make contact with a new self:

I feel proud of myself that I've done something about my vaginismus . . . I feel an enormous relief because the secrecy has gone.

—Sarah

I'm a success story . . . I'm glad I took the help that was available.

—Debbie

Chapter 8

CONCLUSION

I end where I began, by saying that I feel more open and more in touch with who I am. The profound but slow changes which have taken place have occurred in three distinct, yet connected, areas of my life:

- My sexual relationship with my lover. All growth is painful. Because of the vaginismus, my husband and I were forced to make contact with the undeveloped aspects of ourselves which shaped our mutual interactions. We had to grieve over and let go of our past relationship, the "dance" which had created a brother-sister marriage. As we discovered what blocked us from achieving what we truly wanted, new aspects of ourselves started to emerge. We began to understand that a true acceptance of our own and each other's individuality and separateness is the only foundation on which a mature, sexual relationship can be based and real love can grow. Only then could we begin to create a space in which we could give and receive sexually from one another.

- My relationship with my parents. Therapy gave me the ability to view my parents in an objective and multidimensional way. It helped me to recognize and accept that every one of us has our limitations and boundaries. In feeling stronger I was able, although the ability was much delayed, to separate from my mother psychologically. This allowed me to see that her failures were not the result of my "badness" or her inability to love me, but rather the result of the psychological conflicts and social constraints which are universal to many first-time mothers.

The point at which my vaginismus became "fixed" was during the phase in my development when I felt painfully excluded from my parents' shared intimacies and saw that I could not do things with my father that my mother—and other adult women—could. Through therapy I came to understand this and work through it. My persecutory imaginings lost their strength and emotional intensity because I was able to separate fantasy from fact: the baby I had been from the adult I was now. Healing my relationship with my mother and father has been the most powerful part of the reparative process, since the origins of my vaginismus were rooted in that primary relationship.

• My relationship with myself. Because of the growth which took place in the above two areas, my undeveloped self has been able to mature. I no longer experience the world as split, either a blissful or a terrifying place. Instead, the unintegrated parts of me (having to separate my emotions from my body, a confusion about where I end and others begin) have been slowly unified. For the first time the Linda who is me is a whole person with a sense of selfhood and an emotional life of her own.

Like everyone, I have my ups and downs, but on the whole I feel happier and more hopeful about my future. The desperation, alienation and isolation which so haunted me have become much less. My ability to look at and understand what goes on inside me, my husband and family has also helped my relationships with friends. Very few emotional situations feel overwhelming.

In the early hours of Sunday, June 10, 1990, I attended the birth of my friend's baby. It was one of the most profound and moving experiences in my life. Witnessing that birth has helped to heal not only my own birth trauma, but also my fears surrounding my vagina and my feelings of exclusion from an adult, sexual world.

I believe I have come a long way from that toddler who screamed when sand touched her bare feet—not simply in years, but in real growth. My defenses against love and interdependence, and my attempts to hide my needs, are now in the open. I believe these are the final issues I need to understand and work through.

While I have always felt able to feel and express love for others, it is only now that I am beginning to feel love for myself . . . enough love at last to understand and heal my vaginismus. But the end of my story is really the beginning, because the journey to become myself, free and autonomous, goes on.

AFTERWORD

16th July 1990

P.O. Box 820
London N10 3AW

Dear Linda (Valins),

I read your book. Thank you at last for *one* book, one whole
book on vaginismus. I only discovered its existence through
a catalog of Ashgrove Press, which I had due to trying to
find publications on depression. For years I sort of "knew"
about my vaginismus—I couldn't believe a whole book
on it!

Reading your book really put me in touch with how the
problem has affected me and my life, the loneliness, the depression, the "block"—as you call it—from all areas of life: career,
hobbies, friends, relationships. Reading the stories of the
women in your book—and of yourself—made me cry as I've
never been able to cry before, with relief, sadness and hope.

I am writing to you now as a result of your suggesting
support groups in the back of your book. I would very much
like to be in contact with other women, both to help and be
helped. When I think about my life I know I am terrified of
intimacy (not only physical) and yet I don't want to be alone
for the rest of my life.

I am so grateful to you, and would love to get involved
and help others one day.

Yours sincerely,
Naomi

Naomi's letter is one of hundreds I have received since my book was published, and I cannot express what a privilege it is to have women entrust me with their private pain. It takes enormous courage to write to a stranger, and I acknowledge and thank all the women who have taught me so much.

Since its first publication, in England, my book has generated interest and publicity in the field of vaginismus. Two London newspapers (the *Times* and the *Independent*) interviewed me, and I wrote a piece for the *Independent*'s health page, as well as articles for twelve women's magazines. Five national radio talk shows invited me onto their programs, and I appeared on national and cable TV three times (twice in 1989 and once in 1990). I cannot personally take credit for bringing vaginismus to the consciousness of so many. Ideas only come through a person because they are ready to be revealed and heard, and vaginismus was ready to reveal itself. My book just happened to be a vehicle which allowed that to take place.

Although I was prepared to hear from vaginismus sufferers, I was totally unprepared for the many letters I received from women suffering from gynecological and other related conditions. These women felt there was no one else to turn to, indicating a need for increased awareness and sensitivity in the field of gynecology.

More physicians are becoming receptive to the fact that if women are silenced they are forced to express distress through their bodies, and an awareness of vaginismus and its origins has led to the surfacing of other conditions. Recent articles report on *vulvodynia* (also known as *vulval papillomatosis*), genital pain that is an unspoken source of torment for many women. I hope that such related conditions will also be sensitively addressed.

Because I am British, there are bound to be differences in my culture and experiences from those of American women. However, I try to be aware of the sensitive issues of color, culture, race and religion. I have noticed that where there is extreme poverty and oppression, the vaginismus may remain hidden and may be more difficult for a sufferer to reveal.

Although I live in London, which may seem a world apart from the vastness of the United States, the essence of my book and the pain and origins of our vaginismus are universal to all women, wherever we live.

With love,

Linda Valins
London
February 1992

APPENDIX:

WHERE ARE THE

TREATMENTS AVAILABLE?

Treatments for vaginismus are available within both public and private medicine. However, because sexual problems and psychotherapy in general tend not to be given high priority, waiting lists in public health agencies may be long, and the time allocated to a woman may fall short of what is necessary. If treatment is not available or is not satisfactory in public agencies, a woman should not be deterred from seeking help privately. While such treatment is not free, fees are often negotiable depending on financial circumstances.

The term "psychosexual," used in the context of treating vaginismus, simply describes a method concerned with the psychological as opposed to physical aspects of sex, though it appears to be an umbrella term used to describe various methods of treating sexual problems and may not define any one method.

Most private therapies tend to be based mainly in the large cities, and waiting lists are generally shorter than those at public health agencies. I hope that as the need for psychotherapy becomes more generally acknowledged access to private facilities will become more widespread.

Though I am unable to personally recommend any particular doctor, clinic or treatment, I hope you will use my suggestions as a guide. As explained in Chapter Four, I believe it is always advisable to contact therapists through professional associations, thus ensuring that they are members of recognized bodies and thereby governed by standards of professional ethics.

THE PRIMARY CARE PHYSICIAN

While most family doctors are sympathetic, it should be recognized that the majority are not sufficiently trained, nor do they have the time, to offer treatment for vaginismus themselves. You may, of course, be one of the lucky ones whose physician has undertaken some special sexual training or perhaps is a medical hypnotist or has counseling skills. If so, he or she will be able to offer you treatment, providing you wish to work with him or her.

The advantage of treating vaginismus at the primary care level is that it can be dealt with when it first appears, before it is reinforced. For example, vaginismus may first appear in a young woman asking for contraception. If the physician has difficulties in giving her a Pap test, he should be able to recognize her condition and explore it with her. As Dr. Martin Weisberg, M.D., has written, referring to behavioral techniques:[1]

> If there are not substantial underlying interpersonal or intrapsychic problems, there is no reason why a primary care physician could not do (this type of) therapy. . . .

As health systems in the U.S. move away from hospital-based services toward more community–based primary care facilities, centers funded under Health Maintenance Organizations (HMOs) are providing health-care teams under one roof. These often comprise family physicians in association with obstetrical and gynecological departments. It is hoped that this will allow greater cooperation and collaboration between primary care physicians and gynecologists in a non-institutional, local setting.

Since early diagnosis and help with vaginismus can prevent

a woman from seeking inappropriate treatment, I believe it is important that as many family physicians as possible receive training in treating this condition.

As sex therapy training officer Alison Clegg explains, a GP may be a woman's only contact:

> The GP very often can be the first person a woman approaches for help. If a woman receives no help from her GP, she may feel unable ever again to ask for help from anyone else.

However, if your general practitioner is unable to treat you, a consultation with him or her should result in a referral to one of the following:

PSYCHOTHERAPY AND SEXUAL THERAPY IN HOSPITALS AND CENTERS

Many large hospitals and medical centers run sex therapy clinics, and although it varies somewhat, the treatment generally offered is based on a modified version of Masters & Johnson's. Set up on an appointments system, the service is similar to an outpatient clinic. You can also telephone the department of psychology or psychiatry at the nearest major hospital and ask whether the department has a sexual dysfunction or human sexuality clinic, or in the U.K., you can check with your District Health Authority's Department of Clinical Psychology, or with the Family Planning Information Service, 27 Mortimer Street, London W1N 7RJ, tel: 636-7866, and ask for Clinic Enquiries. (See "Human Sexuality/Sexual Dysfunction Programs" on the next page.)

For information about treatment in the U.K., I include an extensive listing of what's available both in the NHS and in private medicine, including professional organizations that make referrals, sex therapy clinics and counselling services, alternative, and complementary treatments and self-help resources.

PROFESSIONAL ORGANIZATIONS AND ASSOCIATIONS THAT
CAN REFER YOU TO A PRACTITIONER IN THE U.S.

In this listing, the more common forms of treatment for
vaginismus appear first.

Human Sexuality/Sexual Dysfunction Programs

Sex counseling services are offered in most major hospitals
and in some medical schools in larger cities. Consult your
family physician, or telephone the departments of psychology, psychiatry, obstetrics and gynecology, or behavioral
medicine at nearby hospitals or medical schools to ask
whether they offer sexual counseling for vaginismus. Any
community hospital will employ a social worker who may
be able to refer you to a therapist or gynecologist in your
area; social workers are generally reliable sources.

Certified Sex Therapists and Counselors

American Association of Sex Educators,
Counselors and Therapists (AASECT)
435 North Michigan Avenue
Suite 1717
Chicago, IL 60611–4067
(312) 644-0828

AASECT publishes a list, available for a small fee, of certified
sex therapists/counselors in each state.

OB/GYN Nurse-Practitioners and Midwives

Physicians and Health Maintenance Organizations (HMOs)
will often hire OB/GYN nurses for their primary health-care
clinics, which are listed in the telephone directory under
"Health Services."
    Alternatively, contact the state nurses' association for cer-

tified nurses and members of the National Association of American OB/GYN Nurses.

Or contact:

Boston Women's Health Book Collective
240A Elm Street
Somerville, MA 02144
(617) 625-0271

The center may be able to refer you to a registered nurse-practitioner known to its staff.

See also the listings for The Maternity Center (page 280) and Nurse-Practitioner Associates (page 281).

Psychodynamic/Psychoanalytic Therapy

National Association for the Advancement of Psychoanalysis and the American Boards for Accreditation and Certification (NAAP)
80 Eighth Avenue
Suite 1210
New York, NY 10011
(212) 741-0515

The NAAP publishes, for a small fee, a National Registry of Psychoanalysts which lists certified practitioners throughout the United States.

See also the listing below for the Women's Therapy Centre Institute.

Feminist Therapy

Women's Therapy Center
80 East 11th Street
Suite 101
New York, NY 10003
(212) 420-1974

The center can make referrals to therapists in the New York area (and some outside it) who are sympathetic to women's psychological and social issues.

Marital and Family Therapy

American Association for Marriage and Family Therapy
1100 17th Street NW
10th Floor
Washington, DC 20036
(202) 452-0109

The association makes referrals free of charge to qualified marriage and family therapists throughout the United States. Write with your Zip Code for a list of therapists which includes a free consumer's guide.

Hypnosis

Institute for Research in Hypnosis and Psychotherapy
1991 Broadway
New York, NY 10023
(212) 874-5290

Write or telephone for a list of certified practitioners.

American Association of Professional Hypnotherapists
P.O. Box 731
McLean, VA 22101
(703) 448-9623

Write or telephone for referrals in your area.

Homeopathic, Alternative and Complementary Practitioners

Homeopathic Educational Services
212 Kittredge Street
Berkeley, CA 94704

National Center for Homeopathy
801 North Fairfax Street
Suite 306
Alexandria, VA 22134

International Foundation for Homeopathy
2366 Eastlake Avenue E
No. 301
Seattle, WA 98102

The above three organizations each publish a directory of homeopaths.

American Holistic Medical Association
4101 Lake Boone Trail No. 201
Raleigh, NC 27607
(919) 787-0116

Members are M.D.s and D.O.s (Doctors of Osteopathy) with a holistic approach to medicine. Send a stamped self-addressed envelope for a referrals list which includes members' complementary specialties.

Taoist Health Institute
(See the listing for Dr. Jing Nuan Wu on page 284.)

Sexuality/Vaginismus Groups

Women's centers in your area may have details. However, as vaginismus is still a relatively new focus, you may have to generate interest yourself by creating a group (see "Self-Help Resources" on page 284).

Institute for Advanced Study of Human Sexuality
1523 Franklin Street
San Francisco, CA 94109
(415) 928-1133

The institute is a private graduate school with a clinical department. It offers a range of services for all kinds of sexual difficulties. Sexuality workshops and all women's groups are run solely by women.

Group Therapy

In general, group therapy is conducted by individual therapists in private practice.

American Group Psychotherapy Association
25 East 21st Street
6th Floor
New York, NY 10010
(212) 477-2677

Members have, at a minimum, a master's degree in a clinical specialty such as psychiatric social work or psychology. When you write or telephone, you will be referred to a local affiliate chapter, which handles referrals to group therapists.

Counseling for Members of Religious and Ethnic Groups

As mentioned before there may well be cultural, religious and ethnic influences which come into play at the onset of vaginismus. In particular it has come to my notice that in cultures where the ritual removal of the clitoris ("clitoridectomy") has been performed the women tend to suffer from a number of problems, including vaginismus. The inclusion of the following contacts is in response to sufferers' requests for counseling and therapy which are sensitive to their culture:

Catholic Charities Families' and Children's Services
2380 Belmont Avenue
Bronx, NY 10458
(212) 364-7700

This agency serves the New York area only. For services in other areas, see under "Catholic Associations" in your local telephone directory.

Indian Health Service Mental Health Program
Special Initiatives Team
300 San Mateo NE
Suite 500
Albuquerque, NM 87108
(505) 766-2873

The program can make referrals to therapists who deal
with particular health issues of the Native American community.

Jewish Board of Children's and Family Services
(212) 582-9100

The board serves the New York area only. For referrals in
other areas, see below.
Association of Jewish Family and Children's Agencies
(908) 821-0909

The association can refer you to the Jewish Family Service
in your area.

Latino Network
32 Rutland Street
Boston, MA 02118
(617) 262-7248

The Latino Network serves as an advocate for the health
needs and rights of the Latino community. Its "Hotline" is
used as a referrals base to connect callers to various sources,
including counselors and therapists.

National Black Women's Health Project
1237 Gordon Street
Atlanta, GA 30310
(404) 753-0917

The project offers self-help groups for black women concerned about health issues. It can also provide referrals for
therapy throughout the United States.

INDIVIDUALS AND CENTERS IN THE U.S.
TREATING VAGINISMUS

The following practitioners have been selected based on personal recommendations to the author by other eminent specialists in the field of vaginismus, and personal contact with the author as a result of published literature. They have kindly agreed to be listed in this book. Again, a listing does not imply a specific recommendation.

Dr. Lonnie Barbach, Ph.D.
341 Spruce Street
San Francisco, CA 94118
(415) 383-0755

Dr. Louanne C. Cole, Ph.D. (Clinical Sexologist)
3025 Fillmore Street
Suite A
San Francisco, CA 94123
(415) 923-9180

Dr. Marian E. Dunn, Ph.D. (Sexologist)
Director
Center for Human Sexuality
State University of New York
Health Science Center
450 Clarkson Avenue
Brooklyn, NY 11203
(718) 270-1750

Professor Julia Heiman, Ph.D. (Clinical Psychologist)
University of Washington
Outpatient Psychiatry Center
Reproductive and Sexual Medicine Clinic
4225 Roosevelt Way NE
Suite 306
Seattle, WA 98105
(206) 543-3555

Dr. Vicki Hufnagel, M.D. (Gynecologist)
Medical Director
Institute for Reproductive Health and Center for Female Re-
constructive Surgery
8721 Beverly Boulevard
Los Angeles, CA 90048
(213) 854-6483

Anita Jordan, Ed.D., A.C.S.
Wadle & Associates P.C. Counseling Services
8230 Hickman Road
Suite B
Des Moines, IA 50325
(515) 270-1344

Dr. Helen Singer Kaplan, M.D., Ph.D.
(Professor of Psychiatry)
30 East 76th Street
4th Floor
New York, NY 10021
(212) 249-2914

See also the listing for New York Hospital–
Cornell Medical Center on page 281.

Dr. Niels Lauersen, M.D. (Obstetrician and Gynecologist)
784 Park Avenue
New York, NY 10021
(212) 744-4222

Marilyn Lawrence, Ed.D. (Sexologist)
1601 Livonia Avenue
Los Angeles, CA 90035
(213) 203-0922

Dr. Sandra Leiblum, Ph.D. (Professor of Clinical Psychiatry)
University of Medicine and Dentistry of New Jersey
Robert Wood Johnson Medical School
675 Hoes Lane
Piscataway, NJ 08854
(201) 463-4273

Dr. Joan Seif Levi, Ph.D., L.C.S.W.
1901 Brickell Avenue
#1813
Miami, FL 33129
(305) 856-9459
also:
2699 Stirling Road
A-105
Ft. Lauderdale, FL 33312
(305) 987-3698

Dr. Carolyn Livingston, R.N., Ph.D.
(Certified Sex Therapist)
Seattle Sexual Health Center
7813 12th Avenue NE
Seattle, WA 98115
(206) 527-8774

Professor Joseph LoPiccolo, Ph.D. (Clinical Psychologist)
Department of Psychology
University of Missouri
Columbia, MO 65211
(314) 882-7752

Dr. William H. Masters, M.D.
(Obstetrician and Gynecologist)
Director
Masters & Johnson Institute
24 South Kingshighway
St. Louis, MO 63108
(314) 361-2377

The Maternity Center
6506 Bells Mill Road
Bethesda, MD 20817
Contact: Marion McCartney, Certified Nurse-Midwife
(301) 530-3300

Dr. Judith A. Meisner, Ph.D.
Counseling and Consulting Services of Pinellas County Inc.
3500 Building
Suite 209
3530 First Avenue North
St. Petersburg, FL 33713
(813) 327-1672

Dr. Carol Nadelson, M.D. (Psychiatrist)
Department of Psychiatry
New England Medical Center Hospitals
750 Washington Street
Boston, MA 02111
(617) 956-6280

New York Hospital–Cornell Medical Center
Human Sexuality Program
Payne Whitney Clinic
525 East 68th Street
New York, NY 10021
(212) 249-2914

This is a part-time program, so all messages are relayed via
Dr. Helen Singer Kaplan's private practice (see listing on page
279)

Nurse-Practitioner Associates
2464 Massachusetts Avenue
Cambridge, MA 02140
Contact: Mimi Clark Secor, Registered Nurse-Practitioner
(617) 354-6028

Dr. Debora Phillips
435 N. Bedford Avenue
#403
Beverly Hills, CA 90210
(213) 278-6342

also:
Princeton Center for Behavior Therapy
211 N. Harrison Street
Princeton, NJ 08540
(609) 924–1212

Professor Kenneth J. Reamy, M.D., M.P.H.
(Professor of Obstetrics and Gynecology, and Behavioral
Medicine and Psychiatry)
Departments of Obstetrics, Gynecology, Behavioral Medi-
cine and Psychiatry
West Virginia University School of Medicine and Medical
Center
Morgantown, WV 26506
(304) 293–5631

Dr. Domeena Renshaw, M.D. (Professor of Psychiatry)
Director
Sexual Dysfunction Clinic
Loyola University Chicago
Loyola University Medical Center
Stritch School of Medicine
2160 South First Avenue
Maywood, IL 60153
(708) 216–3750

Dr. Miriam Rosenthal, M.D. (Psychiatrist)
Department of Obstetrics and Gynecology
MacDonald Hospital for Women
University Hospitals of Cleveland
Cleveland, OH 44106
(216) 844–3941

Dr. Judith Seifer, R.N., Ph.D. (Certified Sex Therapist)
P.O. Box 147
Dayton, OH 45409
(513) 435–3280

Dr. Leslie R. Schover, Ph.D. (Staff Psychologist)
and Dr. David M. Youngs, M.D. (Gynecologist)
Center for Sexual Function (Desk A100)
Cleveland Clinic Foundation
One Clinic Center
Cleveland, OH 44195-5041
(216) 444-3770

Dr. Patricia Schreiner-Engel, Ph.D.,
and Dr. Georgia H. Witkin, Ph.D.
Psychological Services of the Obstetrics and Gynecology
Department
Mt. Sinai Medical Center
1176 5th Avenue (Box 1170)
New York, NY 10029
(212) 241-1726

Dr. Sharen Shapiro, Ph.D., M.F.C.C.
9531 Sepulveda Boulevard
#2
Sepulveda, CA 91343
(818) 893-8509

Professor John F. Steege, M.D. (Gynecologist),
and Dr. Anna L. Stout, Ph.D. (Clinical Psychologist)
Box 3263
Duke University Medical Center
Durham, NC 27710
(919) 684-5322

Dr. Libby A. Tanner, Ph.D., L.C.S.W., L.M.F.T.
5901 S.W. 100 Terrace
Miami, FL 33156
(305) 665-4934

Dr. Leonore Tiefer, Ph.D.
(Clinical Associate Professor, Departments of Urology and Psychiatry)
Department of Urology
Montefiore Medical Center/
Albert Einstein College of Medicine
111 East 210th Street
Bronx, NY 10467-2490
(212) 920-4576

Dr. Judyth O. Weaver, Ph.D.
(Somatic Psychologist/Reichian-based Awareness Therapist)
73 Montford Avenue
Mill Valley, CA 94941
(415) 388-3151

Dr. Jing Nuan Wu, OMD
(Oriental Medical Doctor & Acupuncturist)
Taoist Health Institute
2141 Wisconsin Avenue NW
Washington DC 20007
(202) 265-1603

SELF-HELP RESOURCES (U.S.)

Groups

Even during therapy, there may be times when a woman feels isolated and despairing. While these feelings can, of course, be explored with a therapist, they may nonetheless remain painful reminders of the sense of exclusion from the sexually active world. Because many of us—including me— have suffered alone, the importance of meeting others cannot be overestimated. The suggestions below are not exhaustive, and I hope they lead to further ideas and contacts:

- Place cards or flyers in local feminist bookshops, women's centers and health clinics indicating your interest in meeting other women and starting a self-help support group.

- Write articles or letters for publication in feminist magazines and women's health newsletters asking other sufferers to contact you.

To ensure that you make contact with women who understand what vaginismus is and are genuine sufferers, it may
be helpful to briefly describe the symptoms. You may wish
to use a post-office box number instead of your home address
or telephone number to protect your privacy and security.

Workshops, groups, information and advice on self–help
related to vaginismus may be offered by:
Women's Therapy Center
See listing on page 273.

Boston Women's Health Collective
See page 273.

Vancouver Women's Health Collective
Le Collectif de la Santé des Femmes de Vancouver
Suite 302
1720 Grant Street
Vancouver, BC
V5L 2Y7 Canada
(604) 255-8285

As explained on page 217, a support group for vaginismus
sufferers was established in the United Kingdom in April
1990. Its membership is open to, and welcomes, women from
the United States. For further details write, enclosing an International Reply Coupon, to:

Resolve
P.O. Box No. 820
London N10 3AW
England

Other Resources

Medical literature and other publications on the subject of
vaginismus may be obtainable from the women's health col-
lectives listed on page 272 and above, since they maintain
their own libraries and publish information on women's
health issues.

You can also buy or rent a video available titled "Treating
Vaginismus," which shows a couple going through a treatment program. This tape may be a valuable resource for you
and your partner, but it is advisable to first discuss it with
your doctor or therapist. The video is available from:

Focus International
14 Oregon Drive
Huntington Station, NY 11746
(800) 843-0305

Professional Organizations and Associations That Can Refer You to a Practitioner in the U.K.

Institute of Psychosexual Medicine
11 Chandos Street
Cavendish Square
London W1M 9DE
Tel: 071-580 0631

Members are doctors who have been specifically trained to
develop their skills to treat vaginismus and other psychosexual problems. They have been approved by a panel at the
institute. Upon request and receipt of a stamped addressed
envelope a list of doctors in your area will be forwarded,
including those who practice in the NHS and privately. However, if you wish to telephone for details, a staff member of
the institute is available on the telephone between 9.00 A.M.
and 3.00 P.M. Thursdays only.

Association of Sexual & Marital Therapists
P.O. Box 62
Sheffield S10 3TS
Tel: 0742-303901

Promotes standards of therapy, training, and research into
marital and sexual problems. Members come from varied
disciplines of psychology, medicine, counselling, nursing and
education. Upon receipt of a stamped addressed envelope, a
list of NHS and private clinics in your area will be forwarded
to you.

The Tavistock Clinic
120 Belsize Lane
London NW3 5BA
Tel: 071-435 7111

This is an NHS unit so treatment is free, but the area the
clinic serves is limited to North London and North East
Thames Region only. Psychotherapy as opposed to sexual
therapy is generally offered.

Birmingham Women's Counselling & Therapy Centre
43 Ladywood Middleway
Birmingham B16 8HA
Tel: 021-455 8677

Self-referral but jurisdiction is Central Birmingham Health
District only. Offers individual therapy and counselling from
a feminist perspective. Initial assessment offered and treatment is free.

Brook Advisory Centres
Central Office: 153A East Street
London SE17 2SD
Tel: 071-708 1234

Although free, Brook is not part of the NHS.

Self-referral. Service generally offered for women under twenty-five years of age. Some centers impose strict age limits but others don't, so it is best to check first. Generally the service is free but, again, some centers may charge fees for counselling. As well as treatment for sexual problems they provide free birth control. Contact Central Referrals Secretary for details. (See also COUNSELLING, p. 307).

British Association for Counselling
37A Sheep Street
Rugby
Warwickshire CV21 3BX

Registered charity whose aims are to promote awareness of counselling throughout the U.K. and maintain and raise standards of practice. Inquiries cannot be dealt with by telephone, but if you send a stamped addressed envelope, a list of therapists, both in the NHS and private sector will be sent. You may also request a pamphlet entitled "Counselling and Psychotherapy: Is It For Me?," published by the association.

The London Clinic of Psychoanalysis
63 New Cavendish Street
London W1M 7RD
Tel: 071-580 4952/3

Because demand for analysis is greater than the number of available analysts there are only a limited number of sessions available within the NHS or at reduced fees. Because of limited places, there is a careful assessment procedure. Since analysis does not dwell on the symptom, the assessment is not based upon what kind of problem you have but rather a patient's commitment and motivation to attend five times weekly for at least two years. GP may contact clinic directly.

The Medical Advisory Service
10 Barley Mow Passage
London W4 4PH
Tel: 081-994 9874

Help and information-giving charity run 10 A.M.–10 P.M. Monday through Friday by trained nurses, including a gynecological nurse. They will be able to advise on what treatments are available, and where, both in the NHS and in the private sector, including referrals to a specialist.

Women's Health Concern
83 Earl's Court Road
London W8 6EF
Tel: 071-938 3932

Send stamped, addressed envelope on where to receive help for vaginismus.

Women's Health Information & Reproductive Rights Centre
52 Featherstone Street
London EC1Y 8RT
Tel: 071-251 6580

Charity with data banks and computers detailing women's groups nationwide and can advise on most aspects of women's health.

The Good Doctor Guide by Martin Page (London: Sphere, 1989). The first consumer's directory listing some of the top London specialists in various areas of medicine, including gynecology. It only lists London specialists but very often a gynecologist is likely to know of colleagues treating vaginismus ouside London.

Treatment Within the National Health Service, England

The following are establishments with whom I have had contact. However, this list is a summary, and any omissions do not in any way imply the unsuitability of a clinic. If your area is not covered in this section please refer to page 286 for how best to locate your nearest clinic. In addition, I have produced "The Directory of Treatments for Vaginismus," a booklet which can be purchased from Resolve, P.O. Box

820, London N10 3AW. Unless otherwise stated, *it will always be necessary for either your general practitioner or a hospital consultant to refer you*, therefore this is intended purely as a guide for you and your doctor. At the time of writing these clinics were operating but due to closures of many units it is advisable for your doctor to check on current availability.

Important: Please be prepared for long waiting lists: approximately one to six months, and maybe longer in some cases, because only a limited number of patients can be seen due to financial cutbacks and shortages of practitioners.

London

NORTH LONDON

Sexual Problems Clinic
Royal Free Hospital
2nd Floor, Psychiatric Outpatients Department
Pond Street
London NW3 2QG
Tel: 071-794 0500
(Thursday afternoons)

United Elizabeth Garrett Andeson
& Soho Hospital for Women
Psychosexual Clinic
Outpatients Department
144 Euston Road
London NW1 2AP
Tel: 071-387 2501

For psychosexual clinics in Colindale, Edgware, Finchley, Golders Green and Hendon contact the Barnet Health Authority on 081-449 8711.

EAST LONDON

London Hospital Whitechapel (Walk-In Clinic)
The Ambrose King Centre
Turner Street
London E1 1BB
Tel: 071-377 7307

(Initial point of contact then referral to appropriate practitioner)

CENTRAL LONDON

Margaret Pyke Centre (Part of Soho Hospital for Women)
15 Bateman Buildings
Soho Square
London W1V 5TW
Tel: 071-734 9351. Ext: 212

SOUTH LONDON

St. George's Hospital
Outpatients Department
Clare House
Blackshaw Road
London SW17 OQT
Tel: 081-672 1024

Maudsley Hospital
Psychosexual Clinic
Outpatients Department
Denmark Hill
London SE5 9RS
Tel: 071-703 6333. Ext: 2371

Institute of Psychiatry
(Linked with Maudsley Hospital)
Clinical Services
De Crespigny Park
London SE5 8AF
Tel: 071-703 5411

WEST LONDON

Department of Psychology
Charing Cross Hospital
(Part of West London Hospital)
Fulham Palace Road
London W6 8RF
Tel: 081-846 1234

GREATER LONDON

Psychosexual Counselling Clinic
Caryl Thomas Clinic
Headstone Dive
Wealdstone
Middx HA1 4UQ
Tel: 081-863 7004

Department of Clinical Psychology
Northwick Park Hospital
Watford Road
Harrow
Middx HA1 3UJ
Tel: 081-869 2325/6

Outside London

SOUTH REGIONS:

Hove District Psychology Service
11 Rutland Gardens
Hove BN3 4AG
Tel: 0273-778383. Ext: 158

Psychosexual & Marital Difficulties Clinic
Family Planning Clinic
Avenue House
The Avenue
Eastbourne
Sussex BN21 3XY
(Referrals in writing only)

Psychosexual Clinic
Day Unit Buccleuch House
102 Carisbrooke Road
Newport
Isle of Wight PO30 1DB
Tel: 0983-525254

The Island Clinical Psychology Service
Whitecroft
Sandy Lane
Newport
Isle of Wight PO30 3EB
Tel: 0983-526011. Ext: 250

(Can advise on availability, if any, of other IOW clinics)

Psychosexual Clinic
Central Health Clinic
East Park Terrace
Southampton SO9 4WN
Tel: 0703-634321. Ext: 210

(Self-referral).

East Surrey Psychology Service
Tandridge Day Unit
Caterham Dene Hospital
Church Hill
Caterham-on-the-Hill CR3 5RA
Tel: 0883-47373

Family Planning/Psychosexual Clinic
Baltic Road
Tonbridge
Kent
Tel: 0732-352015

(Self-referral)

District Psychology Service
Farnham Road Hospital
Guildford
Surrey GU2 5LX
Tel: 0483-571122. Ext: 2630

The Help for Health Trust

RESOURCES:

Highcroft Cottage
Romsey Road
Winchester SO22 5DH
Tel: 0962-849079 & 0962-849100 (Answerphone)

(Information service for health care staff and consumers on availability of health services, self-help groups and literature to the people of Hampshire and the Isle of Wight area). The director of The Help for Health Trust has also written a helpful guide for consumers of health services, including help-lines titled *The Health Care Consumer Guide* by Robert Gann (London: Faber & Faber, 1991).

East Regions

Clinical Psychology Services
Shrodells Unit
Watford General Hospital
Vicarage Road
Watford WD1 8HB
Tel: 0923-217441

Psychology Department
Essex County Hospital
Lexden Road
Colchester CO3 3NB
Tel: 0206-853535. Ext: 4605

(Self-referral but it will be necessary for your GP to contact
this department subsequently with his permission)

Community Mental Health Team
90 East Hill
Colchester CO1 2QN
Tel: 0206-761901. Ext: 36

(Team staffed by community psychiatric nurses, a psychologist, as well as staff who are interested in sexual problems)

Psychosexual Clinic
Liverpool Road Health Centre
9 Mersey Place
Luton LU2 7AY
Tel: 0582-424133

(Monday mornings, Wednesday mornings and Thursday
afternoons)

Ipswich Psychosexual Clinic
St. Clements Hospital
Foxhall Road
Ipswich IP3 8LS
Tel: 0473-715111. Ext: 217

Norfolk Clinical Psychology Services
Gorsefield
250 Drayton High Road
Drayton
Norwich NR8 6BH
Tel: 0603-424222. Ext: 356 or 382

Psychosexual Clinic
Clinic Six/Family Planning
Addenbrookes Hospital
Hills Road
Cambridge CB2 2QQ
Tel: 0223-216321 or 216410

District Clinical Psychology Service
Farthing House Counselling Centre
Farthing Grove
Netherfield
Milton Keynes MK6 4HH

(Referrals in writing only)

West Regions

Psychiatric Department
The Warneford Hospital
Warneford Lane
Headington
Oxford OX3 7JX
Tel: 0865-741717/226262

(Very small service limited to people within this health district. If sufferers from outside are referred, then their health district manager has to agree to pay the Oxfordshire Health Authority for any treatment received).

The Convenor
Couples Clinic
Department of Clinical & Community Psychology
Church Lane
Heavitree
Exeter EX2 5SH
Tel: 0392-411611

Clinical Psychology Services
Psychology Department
Barrow Hospital
Barrow Gurney
Bristol BS19 3SG
Tel: 0275-392811

(Initial assessment only and then referral)

Sex Therapy Clinic
The Laurels
9 Powderham Road
Newton Abbot
Devon TQ12 1EU
Tel: 0626-51925

Joint Therapy Clinic
Nuffield Clinic
Lipson Road
St. Judes
Plymouth PL4 8NQ
Tel: 0752-669709

Cheltenham Family Planning Services
Hospital Site
St. Pauls Road
Cheltenham
Glos GL50 4BW
Tel: 0242-513260 & 521362

Psychosexual Clinic
Held at Somerleigh Clinic
Dorset County Hospital
Princes Street
Dorchester DT1 1TS
Tel: 0305-263123. Ext: 147

Psychosexual Clinics
Family Planning Service
Part of Cornwall Community Health Care Trust
4 St. Clement Vean
Tregolls Road
Truro
Cornwall TR1 1NR
Tel: 0872-74242. Ext: 7051

(Psychosexual clinics in Truro administered from this office)

RESOURCES:

The Help for Health Trust
Highcroft Cottage
Romsey Road
Winchester SO22 5DH
Tel: 0962-849079 & 0962-849100 (Answerphone)

Information service for health care staff and consumers on availability of health services, self-help groups and literature to the people of Dorset, Wiltshire and the Bath area.

Midlands Region

Psychosexual Clinic
% Clinic Three
City Hospital
Hucknall Road
Nottingham NG5 1PB
Tel: 0602-691169. Ext: 45496

Psychosexual Clinic
Dudley Road Hospital
Dudley Road
Birmingham B18 7QH
Tel: 021-554 3801

District Department of Clinical Psychology
North Lincolnshire Health Authority
Baverstock House
County Hospital
Sewell Road
Lincoln LN2 5QY
Tel: 0522-560617

Psychosexual Counselling
Family Planning Unit
Good Hope Hospital
Rectory Road
Sutton Coldfield
West Midlands B75 7RR
Tel: 021-378 2211. Ext: 5191

(For residents of North Birmingham only)

Mental Health Speciality
Department of Psychology
The Psychiatric Unit
Leicester General Hospital
Gwendolen Road
Leicester LE5 4PW
Tel: 0533-490490. Ext: 4767

The Psychosexual Counselling Clinic
Moor Street Clinic
Moor Street
Worcester WR1 3DB
Tel: 0905-21075. Ext: 143

District Clinical Psychology Service
Beechwood House
St. Crispin Hospital
Duston
Northampton NN5 6UN
Tel: 0604-752323. Ext: 2861 or 2862

RESOURCES:

For location of psychosexual clinics in the midlands region, contact: Family Planning Clinic, 5 York Road, Birmingham B16 9HX. Tel: 021-454 8236.

North East Regions

Psychosexual Clinic
Held in Contraception Clinic
Newcastle General Hospital
Westgate Road
Newcastle-on-Tyne NE4 6BE
Tel: 091-273-8811. Ext: 22566

(Thursday mornings)

Psychosexual Clinic
Department of Obstetrics & Gynaecology
Shotley Bridge General Hospital
Consett
Durham DH8 ONB
Tel: 0207-503456

(Wednesday afternoons)

Psychosexual Clinic
Obstetrics & Gynaecology Department
Northern General Hospital
Herries Road
Sheffield S5 7AU
Tel: 0742-434343

Psychosexual Medical Clinic
Family Planning Clinic
29–31 Queens Road
Barnsley
South Yorks S71 1AN
Tel: 0226-730000. Ext: 3657

Psychosexual Clinic
The Clarendon Wing
Leeds General Infirmary
Leeds LS2 9NS
Tel: 0532-432799

Clinic for Psychosexual Disorders
Psychology Department
Clifton Hospital
York YO3 6RD
Tel: 0904-645165

Mental Health Unit
South Tees Psychological Service
Woodlands Road Clinic
Middlesbrough
Cleveland TS1 3BL
Tel: 0642-247311

Laura Mitchell Health Centre
Great Albion Street
Halifax HX1 1YR
Tel: 0422-363541. Ext: 67

North West Regions

'T' Clinic
Royal Liverpool Hospital
Prescot Street
Liverpool L7 8XT
Tel: 051-706 2000

Psychosexual Clinic
Held in Family Planning
Ann Burrow Thomas Health Centre
South William Street
Workington
Cumbria CA14 2ED
Tel: 0900-602244. Ext: 132

Psychosexual Clinic
Hope Hospital
Eccles Old Road
Salford M6 8 HD
Tel: 061-787 4471

Psychosexual Clinic
University Hospital of South Manchester
Psychiatric Unit
Withington Hospital
West Didsbury
Manchester M20 8LR
Tel: 061-447 4436

Psychosexual Team
Halton General Hospital
Nr. Shopping City
Runcorn
Cheshire
Tel: 0928-714567. Ext: 3240

Family Planning Clinic
Alkinson Health Centre
Market Street
Barrow-in-Furness
Cumbria LA14 2LR
Tel: 0229-27212

The Isle of Man

Kingswood House Resource Centre
Harris Terrace
Douglas
Isle of Man
Tel: 0624-625958

Treatments Outside the National Health Service (Private), England

The advantages of private treatment are that you can refer yourself (although in some cases it will be helpful for your doctor to know of the treatment you are receiving) and also that waiting lists are generally much shorter in the private sector.

FINANCIAL CONSIDERATIONS.

Private medical services, unless you have insurance coverage, are becoming increasingly expensive and it may seem daunting to embark on an open-ended treatment. You may also feel it is terribly unjust that not only are you suffering emotionally but you will also have to suffer financially. Individual therapists and counsellors may have negotiable fees and some offer sliding-scale payments.

Your general practitioner is a good place to start since he or she may be able to recommend a clinic, therapist or sensitive gynecologist. If not, you may contact the following directly:

Psychosexual & Sex Therapy

LONDON

Institute of Psychosexual Medicine (details on p. 286).

Association of Sexual & Marital Therapists (details on p. 287).

Relate (formerly National Marriage Guidance Council) Head Office: Herbert Gray College, Little Church Street, Rugby, Warks CV21 3AP. Tel: 0788-573241.

(Offers help for wide range of problems, including vaginismus. At the time of writing Relate has one London branch offering sexual therapy (Central Office, London Marriage Guidance, 76A New Cavendish Street, London W1M 7LB.

Tel: 071–580 1087/8). Fees vary, as do the waiting lists. For other London branches contact the office above. You may also look in local telephone directory for nearest branch, although only the Central Office offers sexual counselling)

Marie Stopes Clinic
Marie Stopes House
108 Whitfield Street
London W1P 6BE
Tel: 071–388 0662/7585

(Registered charity offering services in London, Leeds and Manchester. However, psychosexual counselling is only available at present in London)

London Institute of Human Sexuality
10 Warwick Road
London SW5 9UH
Tel: 071–373 0901

(Offers therapy and counselling for difficulties with relationships including sexual problems)

Outside London

Institute of Psychosexual Medicine (Details on p. 286).

Association of Sexual & Marital Therapists (Details on p. 287).

Relate Head Office: See previous page.

(Offers help for wide range of problems, including vaginismus. At the time of writing Relate has approximately 110 branches nationwide offering sexual therapy. Fees vary, as do waiting lists. For your nearest branches in England, Wales, and Northern Ireland contact office above. You may also look in local telephone directory for nearest branch, although it will not indicate whether the branch offers sexual counselling.

South Regions

BUPA Medical Centre
BUPA Hospital
Bartons Road
Havant
Hants PO9 5NP
Tel: 0705-454511

East Regions

BUPA Medical Centre
Hartswood Hospital
Warley Road
Brentwood CM13 3HR
Tel: 0277-232525

(Not all BUPA centers offer psychosexual counselling, so check first)

BUPA Medical Centre
BUPA Hospital
Heathbourne Road
Bushey
Watford WD2 1RD
Tel: 081-950 9090

(Not all BUPA centers offer psychosexual counselling, so check first)

BUPA Medical Centre
Old Watton Road
Colney
Norwich NR4 7TA
Tel: 0603-505011

West Regions

BUPA Medical Centre
4 Priory Road
Clifton
Bristol BS8 1TY
Tel: 0272-731433

Midlands Region

Institute for Sex Education & Research
40 School Road
Moseley
Birmingham B13 9SN
Tel: 021-449 0892

(Non-profit making company which promotes education, research and therapy in the field of human sexual behavior)

BUPA Medical Centre
Clawson Lodge
403 Mansfield Road
Nottingham NG5 2DP
Tel: 0602-622826

North East Regions

BUPA Medical Centre
81 Clarendon Road
Leeds LS2 9PJ
Tel: 0532-436735

North West Regions

Psychosexual Clinic
BUPA Consulting Suite
Russell Road
Whalley Range
Manchester M16 8AJ
Tel: 061-226 0112. Ext: 2574/5

(Ask for Consultant, Psychosexual Therapy)

NOTE:

For private sex therapy in Scotland, Wales, Ireland, and the Channel Isles see pages 325, 329, 330, 332 and 333.

Counselling (Nationwide):

BRITISH ASSOCIATION FOR COUNSELLING.

The Norwich Centre for Personal & Professional
Development
7 Earlham Road
Norwich NR2 3RA
Tel: 0603-617709

(Client-centered counselling, self-referral with some fees negotiable)

The Well–Woman Centre
29 Queens Road
Reading RG1 4AS
Tel: 0734-503157

(Charity staffed by volunteers and founded in 1985 by the Well–Woman Association for West Berkshire. All services are free which include: counselling, consultation with doctor, self-help groups dealing with depression, menopause, PMS, eating disorders, and tranquilizer withdrawal, a library, information file on wide range of health issues. Runs various courses including assertiveness training plus one day health events)

Brook Advisory Centres (for Central Office, see page 287)

Avon Brook Advisory Centre
Tel: 0272-292136

(One of Brook's centers, which does not impose an age limit and offers sexual counselling)

Birmingham Brook Advisory Centre
Tel: 021-455 0491

(Another of Brook's centers, which does not have an age limit. Initial assessment offered and fees negotiable. There are three other branches of Brook in Birmingham, and you will be referred to the appropriate one)

London Brook Advisory Centre
Tel: 071-580 2991

(Psychosexual counselling free to women up to twenty years; from twenty-one to thirty years fees are charged. No residency restrictions, self-referrals)

Milton Keynes Brook Advisory Centre
Tel: 0908-669215

(Free counselling to all women, no age limit. Open Tuesday evenings 5 P.M.–7 P.M. only, with plans to expand in future)

North East Lancashire Brook Advisory Centre
Tel: 0282-416596

(Short-term counselling mainly for women under twenty-five)

Counselling for Members of Religious and Ethnic Groups

There may well be cultural, religious and ethnic influences that come into play with the onset of vaginismus. In particular it has come to my notice that in cultures where the ritual removal of the clitoris (clitoridectomy) has been performed, the women suffer from all sorts of sexual problems, including vaginismus. The inclusion of the following contacts is in response to women's requests for counselling or therapy, which is sensitive to their cultural backgrounds:

Jewish Marriage Council
Headquarters South:
23 Ravenshurst Avenue
London NW4 4EL
Tel: 081-203 6311

Headquarters North:
Levi House
Bury Old Road
Manchester M8 6FT
Tel: 061-740 5764

(Runs confidential counselling service for marital, family and personal problems and is sensitive and understanding of Jewish culture. Working within this particular framework they are able to be aware and sympathetic to the problems which vaginismus may create within a Jewish marriage or relationship. Fees negotiable.)

Catholic Marriage Advisory Council
Headquarters nationwide:
1 Blythe Mews
Brook Green
London W14 OHW
Tel: 071-371 1341

(Counselling for sexual difficulties from a Catholic orientation, but nondogmatic. Fees variable.)

Foundation for Women's Health Research & Development (FORWARD)
38 King Street
London WC2E 8JT
Tel: 071-379 6889

(Offers brief counselling to black women of African origins with particular understanding of clitoridectomy victims)

NAFSIYAT: The Inter-Cultural Therapy Centre
278 Seven Sisters Road
London N4 2HY
Tel: 071-263 4130

(Charity, free treatment to patients in Islington and Bloomsbury only. Fees charged to people living outside of these districts. Offers psychoanalytic therapy paying special attention to all ethnic minorities cultural factors. Self-referrals, but letter required at the first consultation either from a GP, social worker or self.)

Psychotherapy and Psychoanalysis (Nationwide)

British Association of Psychotherapists
121 Hendon Lane
London N3 3PR
Tel: 081-346 1747

(One of the few professional bodies in the U.K. that trains and qualifies psychotherapists according to agreed standards. Consultation offered with experienced psychotherapist to discuss whether it would be an appropriate form of help and treatment. Orientation of therapists is psychoanalytic, covering Freudian, Jungian and Kleinian concepts. Although majority of members are in London they will endeavor to refer you to someone in your area. Fees for regular treatment are negotiated between patient and therapist. Inquiries may be made in writing to the Referrals Secretary, enclosing a stamped, addressed envelope.)

Society of Analytical Psychology
1 Daleham Gardens
London NW3 5TB
Tel: 072-435 7696

(Members trained in analytical psychology, many are doctors. Majority practice in London, but the SAP will try to refer you to someone in your area. To arrange initial assessment, contact Referrals Secretary in writing, enclosing a stamped, addressed envelope.)

The Guild of Psychotherapists
19B Thornton HIll
London SW19 4HU
Tel: 081-947 0730

(Psychoanalytic psychotherapy with some members outside London. The guild operates its own Code of Ethics and training school, and some therapists offer sliding-scale fees.)

Oxford Centre for Human Relations
9 Junction Road
Oxford OX4 2NT
Tel: 0865-717333

(Laingian and Jungian psychotherapy, various forms of social
and emotional support including free group work)

Feminist Psychotherapy and Counselling

LONDON

Women's Therapy Centre
6 Manor Gardens
London N7 6LA
Tel: 071-263 6200.

(Co-founded by therapists Susie Orbach and Luise Eichenbaum in 1976, the center's philosophy is women-oriented,
offering therapy and group workshops from a feminist perspective. To arrange for assessment write to them enclosing
a stamped, addressed envelope.)

London Women's Therapy Network
3 Carysfort Road
London N16 9AA
Tel: 081-855 2410 & 071-249 7846

(Therapy at regular fees, but possible to refer women on low
incomes to trainee therapists at reduced rates.)

Pellin Centre
43 Killyon Road
London SW8 2XS
Tel: 071-622 0148

(Individual therapy and ongoing groups.)

OUTSIDE LONDON

Birmingham Women's Counselling and Therapy Centre (Details on page 287.)

Women's Counselling and Therapy Service
Top Floor
Oxford Chambers
Oxford Place
Leeds LS1 3AX
Tel: 0532-455725

(Therapy in the Leeds Metropolitan district only. Publicly funded, but donations are encouraged and there may be a waiting list. Offers analytic groups, though not specifically for vaginismus.)

Bradford Womens Counselling and Therapy Service
c/o B.T.O.C.,
108 Sunbridge Road
Bradford BD1 2NE
Tel: 0274-725794

(Women-centered art psychotherapy, individual and groups. Free service to women on low incomes with referrals to private therapists where appropriate.)

Brighton Women's Counselling and Therapy Service
The Threshold Unit
79 Buckingham Road
Brighton BN1 3RT
Tel: 0273-749800

(Free and very low cost counselling and psychotherapy, individual and groups. Referrals to private practitioners where appropriate.)

Sheffield Women's Counselling and Therapy Service
210 Chippinghouse Road
Sheffield S7 1DR
Tel: 0742-550415

(Wide range of group therapy on sliding-scale fees. No individual therapy at present, but plans to offer this to women in the future on no or low incomes.)

Group Therapy:

For professional reasons laid down by the General Medical Council I am unable to include the names of doctors offering group analysis. If you wish to take part in such a group please contact me.

Sexuality Groups for Women:

Redwood Women's Training Association
Head Office: 5 Spennithorne Road
Skellow, Doncaster
South Yorkshire DN6 8PF
Tel: 0302-337151

(Provides courses in assertiveness and sexuality, enabling women to find their strengths, grow in confidence and value themselves. The philosophy of Redwood is not competitive and committed to non-sexist and non-racist principles. Sexuality groups run for eight to ten weeks (a two-hour session each week or for one or two full days). A list of names and addresses of groups in your area throughout the United Kingdom will be sent to you by contacting Sue Turner.)

Alternative and Complementary Therapies

As explained in "Hypnotherapy" (page 141) it would not be appropriate to seek out a hypnotherapist per se for vaginismus, but rather the services of a registered physician or clinical psychologist with training in hypnosis. This is because I feel that hypnotherapy, along with other alternative treatments, should not replace medical treatment but rather complement it.

A comprehensive guide to help you find an appropriate practitioner is *The Holistic Network Directory 1991/92* from The Holistic Network, P.O. Box 1447, London N6 5JN. Tel: 081-341 6789.

Other sources:

Institute of Complementary Medicine
21 Portland Place
London W1N 3AF

(If you would like advice on which alternative therapist to choose for vaginismus you may write, enclosing a stamped, addressed envelope, to Information Service, the Institute's referral service.)

British Society of Medical and Dental Hypnosis
42 Links Road
Ashtead
Surrey KT21 2HJ
Tel: 03722-73522

(Membership limited to doctors and dentists only and if you contact the Referrals Secretary a list of practitioners will be forwarded. Letter of referral is always required from your GP.)

British Society of Experimental and Clinical Hypnosis
Dr. Michael Heap
c/o Department of Psychology
Middlewood Hospital
Sheffield S6 1 TP Tel: 0742-852222. Ext: 2140

(Membership limited to doctors, psychologists, dentists and psychotherapists. Contact Dr. Heap enclosing stamped addressed envelope for list of practitioners in your area. Depending on where you live, he may be able to refer you to someone with expertise in treating vaginismus. Letter of referral from GP required.)

British Homeopathic Association
27A Devonshire Street
London W1N 1RJ
Tel: 071-935 2163.

(Lists doctors who practice homeopathic medicine, hospitals and NHS and private clinics)

Society of Homeopaths
47 Canada Grove
Bognor Regis
West Sussex
P021 1DW
Tel: 0243-860678

(Has register of professional homeopaths who have graduated after four years training and six months clinical assessment. Send stamped, addressed envelope for list of nearest practitioners.)

British Medical Acupuncture Society
Newton House
Newton Lane
Lower Whitley
Warrington
Cheshire WA4 41A
Tel: 0925-730727

(Referrals to fully registered medical practitioners with training and experience in acupuncture)

British Holistic Medical Association
179 Gloucester Place
London NW1 6DX
Tel: 071-262 5299

(Please note: only your GP may contact this association.)

Alternative Medicine Clinics

LONDON

The Women's Natural Health Centre
1 Hillside
Highgate Road
London NW5 1QT
Tel: 071-482 3293

(Psychotherapy)

The Whole Woman Clinic: Integrated Health for Women
The Hale Clinic
7 Park Crescent
London W1N 3HE
Tel: 071-631 0156

(Service offered by women, for women, to understand their needs and problems. Holistic practitioners are available as well as sexual counselling to couples. Fees negotiable.)

Lady Wellcare Clinic
144 Harley Street
London W1N 1AH
Tel: 071-935 0023 & 0344-28383

(Holistic Obstetrician & Gynecologist)

Jeyrani Health Centre
4-6 Glebelands Avenue
London E18 2AB
Tel: 081-580 1146

(Alternative Obstetrician & Gynecologist)

Holistic Healing Practice
27 Westbury Road
London N12 4NY
Tel: 081–446 4854

(Analytical psychotherapy plus range of alternative therapies)

The Naturopathic Private Clinic for Women
11 Alderton Crescent
London NW4 3XU
Tel: 081–202 6242

(Naturopathic investigation and treatment for causes of vaginismus)

Homeopathy for Women
47 Rasper Road
London N20 OLU.
Tel: 081–446 3339

(Homeopathy and counselling, with special interest in women and children)

Positive Health Centre
101 Harley Street
London W1N 1DF
Tel: 071–935 3858

(Holistic medical practitioner, sliding-scale fees)

Outside London

The Natural Health Clinic
149 Elgar Avenue
Surbiton
Surrey KT5 9JX
Tel: 081–399 9022

(Naturopathic approach to vaginismus and gynecological problems, including acupuncture and osteopathy)

The Bournemouth Centre of Complementary Medicine
26 Sea Road
Boscombe
Bournemouth
Dorset BH5 1DF
Tel: 0202-396354

(Wide range of alternative therapies, including medical doctors)

The Minster Centre
15 Silver Street
Ilminster
Somerset TA19 ODH
Tel: 0460-57930

(Holistic counselling/therapy/hypnotherapy)

Bretforton Hall Clinic
Bretforton
Vale of Evesham
Worcestershire WR11 5JH
Tel: 0386-850537

(Alternative medical practitioners)

Homeopathic Health Clinic
29 Streatfield Road
Kenton Middx HA3 9BP
Tel: 081-907 4885

(Consulting physician in homeopathic medicine)

The Surgery
20 Drury Road
Colchester
Essex CO2 7UX
Tel: 0206-575581

(Homeopathic medical practitioner)

Gateways Centre
Blackhorse Road
Woking GU22 ORE
Tel: 0483-23203

(Psychotherapist with background in complementary medicine, using natural remedies—(herbal, homeopathic, vita-
mins and minerals)—to support the therapy when necessary)

Self-Help Resource Guide

Even during therapy there may be times when we feel isolated
and lonely. While these feelings can, of course, be explored
and shared with our thearpist they may nonetheless remain
painful reminders of our sense of exclusion from the sexually-
active world. Because many of us, including me, have suffered alone, I realize the importance of meeting other sufferers. I have therefore put together some suggestions of places
to contact. The list is not exhaustive and centers mainly on
London, but I hope it may lead to further contacts closer to
home. Not all suggestions relate to self-help groups, but more
to general health-related issues concerning women.

Birmingham Women's Counselling and Therapy Centre

(Details on page 287)
As well as a counselling service they will initiate the setting
up of a self-help group if requested.

National Association for the Childless

Birmingham Settlement, 318 Summer Lane, Birmingham
B19 3RL. Tel: 021-359 4887/2113,
Registered charity and self-help organization for childless
people, concerned with the feelings of those who can't have
children. The NAC helps with the various problems en-

countered by the infertile and although vaginismus does not cause medical infertility it can nevertheless result in childlessness. Send small contribution for membership and stamped, addressed envelope for self-help group in your area. NAC also publishes a newsletter offering information and anecdotes.

Winvisible (Women with Visible and Invisible Disabilities)

King's Cross Women's Centre, 71 Tonbridge Street, London WC1H 9DZ. Tel: 071-837 7509.
WinVisible is a network of black and white women with visible and invisible disabilities, and a member of the International Wages for Housework Campaign. They are campaigning for economic independence, political and social autonomy, mobility, access and housing, against welfare cuts, racism, rape and military-industrial pollution. If you are able to form a local self-help group and need meeting space then WinVisible would be happy to discuss your requirements with the author. Please contact me first via the publisher.

Women's Counselling and Therapy Service

(Details on page 312)
Offers initial advice only to set up a self-help group.

Women and Medical Practice

40 Turnpike Lane, London N8 OPS. Tel: 081-888 2782.

Women's health collective committed to campaigning against all forms of oppression, which may be encountered in the course of medical treatments. As well as offering one-to-one counselling they provide a list of alternative practitioners and a register of local and national women's centers, women's groups and health-related organizations. Would be a valuable contact for self-help group or workshop since one of their members might be prepared to take part in the group. Runs newsletter.

Women's Therapy Centre

(Details in on p. 311).

Offers workshops, group and advice on self-help covering all women's issues. Two vaginismus workshops have been held; one during autumn 1983 and the other on March 26, 1984.

Further suggestions for creating self-help and support groups:

- Place cards and flyers in local feminist bookshops, women's centers and health clinics indicating your interest in meeting other women and starting a self-help/support group.
- Write article or letter for publication in feminist magazines and women's health newsletters requesting other sufferers to contact you.

Note:

To ensure that you make contact with women who understand what vaginismus is and are genuine sufferers, it may be helpful to describe the symptoms briefly. You may also wish to use a post office box number in preference to your home address or telephone number to protect your privacy and security.

Resolve: The Vaginismus Support Group

As explained earlier a support group for vaginismus sufferers was established in the United Kingdom in April 1990. Its membership is open to, and welcomes, all women. For further details send stamped, addressed envelope to:

Resolve
P.O. Box 820
London N10 3AW

Other Resources

FILMS

Vaginismus is featured in two videos called *Female Sex Disorders* and *Sex Disorders: An Introduction*. They are available for rent or purchase from the address below. However, it is advisable to discuss this with your doctor or therapist first.

Dr. Martin Cole
The Institute of Sex Education and Research
40 School Rd.
Moseley
Birmingham B13 9SN
Tel: (021) 449-0892

INFORMATION

Medical literature and other publications on the subject of vaginismus may be obtainable from the various health organizations listed in this section since they maintain their own libraries and publish information on women's health issues.

Women's Centers

Workshops, groups, information and advice on self-help, including publications and literature on vaginismus, may be offered by women's centers nationwide. I have established that the specific resources offered by some centers to vaginismus sufferers are:

- brief counselling
- referrals to female therapists and feminist doctors
- free or rentable space for group meetings
- assistance in setting up a group

However, due to insufficient funding, the future for many of these centers is uncertain. A useful publication, which lists women's centers nationwide is *The Everywoman Directory*, published every May by Everywoman Publishing Ltd. It is available by mail from: Everywoman Sales, 34 Islington Green, London N1 8DU.

Treatment Outside England

SCOTLAND, WITHIN THE NATIONAL HEALTH SYSTEM

Edinburgh Human Sexuality Group
% Marriage Counselling Scotland
26 Frederick Street
Edinburgh EH2 2JR

(Contact: Mrs. Eira Hamilton).
(For referrals to therapists and gynecologists write to the above enclosing a stamped, addressed envelope.)

Lothian Health Board Family Planning/Well Woman Service
The Dean Terrace Centre
18 Dean Terrace
Edinburgh EH4 1NL
Tel: 031-332 7941

Sexual Problems Clinic
% Andrew Duncan Clinic
Morningside Place
Royal Edinburgh Hospital
Edinburgh EH10 5HF
Tel: 031-447 2011

Sexual Dysfunctions Clinic
% Gynaecological Out Patients Dept
Royal Infirmary of Edinburgh
Lauriston Place
Edinburgh EH3 9YW
Tel: 031-229 2477

(Referrals in writing only)

Sexual Dysfunctions Clinic
Department of Psychiatry
Western General Hospital
Crewe Road
Edinburgh EH4 2XU

(Referrals in writing only)

Consultant Gynaecologist
Sexual Dysfunction Clinic
Eastern General Hospital
Seafield Street
Edinburgh EH6 7LN
Tel: 031-554 4444

(Referrals in writing only)

Family Planning Centre
2 Claremont Terrace
Glasgow G3 7XR
Tel: 041-332 9144

Psychosexual Clinic
Carswell House
5 Oakley Terrace
Glasgow G31 2HX
Tel: 041-554 6267 & 556 5222

Family Planning Clinic
Community Health Services
13 Golden Square
Aberdeen AB1 1RH
Tel: 0224-642711

Family Planning Clinic
Loughborough Road
Kirkcaldy
Fife KY1 3DB
Tel: 0592-52133

Psychosexual Clinic
Psychiatric Out Patients Department
Area 3A
Ninewells Hospital
Dundee DD1 9SY
Tel: 00382-60111. Ext: 2742

Scotland, Outside the National Health Service

Marriage Counselling Scotland (Scottish equivalent of Relate)
Headquarters: 26 Frederick Street
Edinburgh EH2 2JR
Tel: 031-225 5006

(There are local councils in Aberdeen, Edinburgh, Glasgow,
Jedburgh and Stirling providing sex therapy. Write or telephone for nearest branch offering such counselling.)

BUPA Medical Centre
Murrayfield Hospital
122 Corstophine Road
Edinburgh EH12 6UD
Tel: 031-334 0363

(Not all BUPA centers offer psychosexual counselling, so
check first)

BUPA Medical Centre
Axton House
295 Fenwick Road
Giffnock
Glasgow G46 6UH
Tel: 041-638 4445

Edinburgh Brook Advisory Centre
50 Gilmore Place
Edinburgh EH3 9NY
Tel: 031-229 3596

(As well as contaceptive services, this center offers psycho-sexual counselling. For further information about the Brook Advisory Centres, see page 287.)

Scottish Institute of Human Relations
56 Albany Street
Edinburgh EH1 3ZR
Tel: 031-556 0924

and: 21 Elmbank Street
Glasgow G2 4PE
Tel: 041-204 3365

(Offers psychoanalytic psychotherapy and counselling)

The Centre of Light
Tighnabruaich
Struy by Beauly
Inverness-shire IV4 7JU
Tel: 046376-254

(Various complementary therapies with intensive one-to-one sessions in countryside setting. For more about alternative medicine, see page 316.)

Resources

Women Unlimited
4A Downfield Place
Edinburgh
Tel: 031-337 5543

Health Help For All
22B McLeod Street
Edinburgh EH11 2NH
Tel: 031-346 8495

(Lending library of books, videos and many leaflets on all aspects of health for both women and men. Informal counselling and referrals.)

Wales (Cymru), within The National Health Service

Cymdeithas Cynllunio Teuluoedd, Gogledd Cymru
Family Planning Association, North Wales
Greenhouse
1 Trevelyan Terrace
High Street
Bangor
Gwynedd LL57 1AX
Tel: 0248-352176

(Information and resource center. Does not offer treatment but can refer.)

Cymdeithas Cynllunio Teuluoedd, Caerdydd, Cymru
Family Planning Association, Wales
6 Windsor Place
Cardiff CF1 2BX
Tel: 0222-342766.

Clinig Seico-Rywiol, Adran Seiciatreg, Ysbyty Gogledd Cymru
Psychosexual Clinic
Department of Psychiatry
North Wales Hospital
Denbigh
Clwyd LL16 5SS

(Referrals in writing only)

Clinigau Camweighrediad Rhywiol, de Cymru
Sexual Dysfunction Clinics, South Wales
Held at Bridgend General & Glanrhyd Hospitals
Tel: 0656–766100. Ext: 2005

Clinig Priodasol Seico-Rywiol
Marital Psychosexual Clinic
Glan Clwyd Hospital
Bodelwyddan
Clwyd
Tel: 0745–583910

Clinig Seico-Rywiol
Psychosexual Clinic
Community Hospital
Hesketh Road
Colwyn Bay
Tel: 0492–515218

Clinig Priodasol/Seico-Rywiol
Ysbyty Dydd
Marital/Psychosexual Clinic
Day Hospital
Royal Alexandra Hospital
Rhyl
Tel: 0745–55188. Ext: 96

Adran Seicoleg
Ysbyty Dydd Menai
Psychology Department
Menai Day Hospital
Ysbyty Gwynedd
Bangor
Tel: 0248–351177. Ext: 4018

Wales, Outside the NHS

Canolfan Feddygol Gogledd Cymru
North Wales Medical Centre
Queens Road
Craigydon
Llandudno Gwynedd LL30 1UD
Tel: 0492-879031

(Ask for Clinical Psychologist.)

Relate Cymru
Relate Wales
Offers sexual counselling at the following five branches: Cardiff, Colwyn Bay, Dyfed, Gwent and Swansea.

Canolfan Feddygol BUPA
Ysbyty BUPA
BUPA Medical Centre
BUPA Hospital
Croescadarn Road
Pentwyn
Cardiff CF2 7XL
Tel: 0222-735515

(Not all BUPA Centres offer psychosexual counselling, so check first)

Resources

Canolfan Menywod Caerdydd
Cardiff Women's Centre
2 Coburn Street
Cathays
Cardiff CF2 4BS
Tel: 0222-383024

Note: I would like to thank David Bullock, Head of Translation, The Welsh Office, Cardiff, for help with the translation of clinics cited here.

Northern Ireland, Within the National Health Service

Belfast City Hospital
Windsor House
Lisburn Road
Belfast BT9 7AB
Tel: Belfast (0232) 329241

Tyrone Fermanna Hospital
1 Donaghranie Road
Omagh
County Tyrone
Tel: 0662-245211

Northern Ireland, Outside the NHS

Relate: Northern Ireland Marriage Guidance
76 Dublin Road
Belfast BT2 7HP
Tel: Belfast (0232) 323454

(Offers sexual therapy and can also refer to psychosexual clinics in local hospitals, if required)

Catholic Marriage Advisory Council
Cana House
56 Lisburn Road
Belfast BT9 6AF
Tel: Belfast (0232) 233002

Family Planning Association (Northern Ireland Regional Office)
113 University Street
Belfast BT7 1 HP
Tel: Belfast (0232) 325488

FPA Derry Office:
14 Magazine Street
Derry BT48 6HH
Tel: 0504-260016

The Surgery
72 Maryville Park
Lisburn
Belfast BT9
Tel: 0232-662729

(Medical acupuncturist)

The Surgery
18 Killinchy Street
Comber Co. Down
Northern Ireland
Tel: 0247-872727

(Holistic Medical Practitioner)

(For more about alternative medicine, see page 316.)

Redwood Ireland
Tel: 010-3531-2844245

(For details about the Redwood Women's Training Association, see page 313. Contact the above number for information about trainers throughout Northern and Southern Ireland.)

Resources

Falls Women's Centre
149 Mulholland Terrace Falls Road
Belfast BT12 6AF
Tel: Belfast (0232) 327672

(No specialist information or counselling on vaginismus, but can be a contact facility for women wishing to get in touch with local sufferers; premises can be used for meetings.)

Women's Centre
19A North Street Arcade
Belfast BT1 1PA
Tel: Belfast (0232) 231676 & 243363

Southern Ireland

Note: There is no NHS in Southern Ireland.

Marriage Counseling Service (equivalent of Relate)
24 Grafton Street
Dublin
Tel: Dublin (010-3531) 720341.

(Referrals to sex therapists)

Catholic Marriage Advisory Council
All Hallows College
Drumcondra
Dublin 9
Tel: Dublin (010-3531) 371151.

(Able to advise on sexual therapy for vaginismus)

Irish Family Planning Association (IFPA)
Information & Education Office: 36–7 Lower Ormond Quay
Dublin 1
Tel: Dublin (010-3531) 730877 or 725394 and Bookshop: 725366

(Offers general information regarding sex therapy and books on sexual difficulties throughout Southern Ireland)

Irish Family Planning Association South City:
59 Synge Street
Dublin 8
Tel: Dublin (010-3531) 682420

Irish Family Planning Association North City:
5-8 Cathal Brugha Street
Dublin 1
Tel: Dublin (010-3531) 727276

Psychiatric Unit
University College Hospital
Galway
Tel: 010-3539-124222. Ext: 458 & 459

Consultant Psychiatrist
Psychosexual Clinic
St. Patrick's Hospital
St. James's Street
P.O. Box 136 Dublin 8
Tel: Dublin (010-3531) 7755423. Ext: 307

Redwood Ireland
Tel: 010-3531-872727

(For details about the Redwood Women's Training Association, see page 313. Contact the above number for information about trainers throughout Northern and Southern Ireland.)

The Channel Isles

Note: There is no NHS in the Channel Isles. While hospital services are free, all patients have to pay their general practitioners.

JERSEY

Clinical Psychology Department
The General Hospital
St. Helier
Jersey JE2 3QS
Tel: 0534-59000. Ext: 2651 & 2426

Consultant Obstetrician & Gynaecologist
Department of Obstetrics & Gynaecology
The General Hospital
St.Helier
Jersey JE2 3QS
Tel: 0534-59000. Ext: 2907

Relate Jersey
2 St. Mark's Lane
St. Helier
Tel: 0534-53756.

GUERNSEY

The States of Guernsey's Mental Health Services offer psychotherapy and counselling for vaginismus. All referrals for treatment must be via the general practitioner in the first instance. Some doctors' practices have a counsellor specifically to deal with this condition.

Relate Guernsey
5 Smith Street
St. Peter Port
Tel: 0481-23853

NOTES

INTRODUCTION

1. Patricia Gillan, consultant psychologist, interview with author, London, 16 September 1987.

CHAPTER 2:

1. *Dyspareunia: Aspects of Painful Coitus*, ed. Herman Musaph and Ary Haspels (Utrecht: Bohn, Scheltema & Holkema, 1977) 18.
2. Philip M. Sarrel, Lorna J. Sarrel and Carol Nadelson, "Dyspareunia and Vaginismus," in *Treatments of Psychiatric Disorders*, vol. 3, Ed. Harold Lief et al. (American Psychiatric Association, 1989), 3.
3. Joan Woodward, "The Diagnosis and Treatment of Psychosomatic Vulvovaginitis," in *The Practitioner* (Birmingham, England: Brook Advisory Centre, 1981), pp. 1–4. This report describes how vaginitis can be sustained by psychological factors, and states that it is not uncommon for general practitioners to doubt that such symptoms could be psychosomatic. The suggested treatments for psychosomatic vulvovaginitis are similar to those for vaginismus.
4. Willeke Bezemer, "Vaginism: A Women's Problem?" (paper presented at Symposium Rutgers Foundation, Heidelberg, West Germany, June 1987), 3.
5. Musaph and Haspels, *Dyspareunia*, 56.
6. Havelock Ellis, *Studies in the Psychology of Sex*, vol. 3 (New York: Random House, 1900).

7. *A Psycho-analytic Dialogue: The Letters of Sigmund Freud and Karl Abraham 1907–1926*, ed. Hilda C. Abraham and Ernst L. Freud. London: Hogarth Press and the Institute of Psycho-analysis, 1965.

8. Sarrel, Sarrel and Nadelson, "Dyspareunia and Vaginismus," 87.

9. Leonard J. Friedman, *Virgin Wives: A Study of Unconsummated Marriages* (London: Tavistock Publications, 1962), 37.

10. Jeffrey M. Masson, *A Dark Science: Women, Sexuality and Psychiatry in the Nineteenth Century*. Translated by Marianne Loring (New York: Farrar, Straus & Giroux, 1987), 128–138.

11. Lindsay Knight, *Talking to a Stranger* (London: Fontana/Collins, 1986), 261.

12. Sandra R. Leiblum and Lawrence A. Pervin, *Principles and Practice of Sex Therapy* (New York: Guilford Press, 1980), 191.

13. These data were gratefully researched using the computer of Dr. Leonard Friedman in Wellesley, Massachusetts, August 1987.

14. "Morbidity Statistics from General Practice," 35–36. Royal College of General Practitioners, London, 1981–82.

15. *Ibid.*, 35–6.

16. *Ibid.*, 35–6.

17. J. Barnes, "Primary Vaginismus: Part 1, Social and Clinical Features." Dublin: *Irish Medical Journal*. 79(3), March 1986, 59–62.

18. May Duddle, "The Clinical Management of Sexual Dysfunction," Royal College of Obstetricians and Gynecologists, London, 1975, 295–6.

19. *Sun Newspaper*, England. Source: courtesy of Deidre Sanders.

20. Friedman, *Virgin Wives*, 130.

21. Leiblum and Pervin, Principles and Practice of Sex Therapy, 168.

22. William H. Masters and Virginia E. Johnson, *Human Sexual Inadequacy* (Boston: Little, Brown & Co., 1970), 243.

23. Sarrel, Sarrel and Nadelson, "Dyspareunia and Vaginismus," 8.

24. *Ibid.*, 8.

25. *Ibid.*, 11.

26. Masters and Johnson, *Human Sexual Inadequacy*, 245.

27. Helen Singer Kaplan, *The New Sex Therapy: Active Treatment of Sexual Dysfunctions* (New York: Brunner-Mazel, 1974), 460.

28. Leiblum and Pervin, *Principles and Practice of Sex Therapy*, 181–82.

29. *Practice of Psychosexual Medicine*, ed. Katharine Draper (London: John Libbey, 1982), 200.

30. Extract from Ampthill Peerage case taken from *The Law Reports Appeal Cases 1977*, House of Lords, (Official Law Reports Series 1, 77, 578 third para F). Reprinted by kind permission of the Incorporated Council of Law Reporting for England and Wales.

31. Jelto J. Drenth, "Vaginismus and the Desire for a Child," *Journal of Psychosomatic Obstetrics and Gynecology* 9 (March 1988): 125–37.

32. *Ibid.*, 125–37.

33. Draper, *Practice of Psychosexual Medicine*, 200.

34. Drenth, "Vaginismus and the Desire for a Child," 125–37.

35. Friedman, *Virgin Wives*, 72.

36. *Ibid.*, 72.

37. *Ibid.*, 72.

38. *Ibid.*, 72.

39. *Ibid.*, 73.

40. Sarrel, Sarrel and Nadelson, "Dyspareunia and Vaginismus," 16.

CHAPTER 3

1. Leiblum and Pervin, *Principles and Practice of Sex Therapy*, 148–9.

2. Musaph and Haspels, *Dyspareunia*, 30.

3. This paragraph is based on earlier writings undertaken in 1989 with the author's friend and colleague Mary Kingsley, a psychotherapist in private practice in London.

4. Luise Eichenbaum and Susie Orbach, *Understanding Women: A Feminist Psychoanalytic Approach* (New York: Basic Books, 1984), 17.

5. Eric Berne, *A Layman's Guide to Psychiatry and Psychoanalysis* (New York: Simon & Schuster, 1968), 142.

6. As Eichenbaum and Orbach cite it in their book *Understanding*

Women (New York: Basic Books, 1984, 113): "Feminist psychoanalysts diverge from the Object Relations Theorists in that they acknowledge that mother is not an 'object' but also a person who is a social and psychological being. What becomes internalized from this perspective isn't then the object, but the different aspects of mother. Object Relations Theorists fail to take into account the psychology of the mother and the effect of the social position of women on that mother's psychology."

7. Susie Orbach, *Hunger Strike: The Anorectic's Struggle as a Metaphor for Our Age* (New York: Avon Books, 1988), 88–9.

8. The Oedipal stage of development, as most people know, was named by Sigmund Freud after the figure from Greek myth who unknowingly killed his father and married his mother.

9. Musaph and Haspels, *Dyspareunia*, 29.

10. Sarrel, Sarrel and Nadelson, "Dyspareunia and Vaginismus," 7.

11. *Dyspareunia*, Musaph and Haspels, 29.

12. Kaplan, *The New Sex Therapy*, 459.

13. Clara M. Thompson, *On Women* (New York: Basic Books, 1971), 136–7.

14. Musaph and Haspels, *Dyspareunia*, 31.

15. Eichenbaum and Orbach, *Understanding Women*, 78–9.

16. Musaph and Haspels, *Dyspareunia*, 32.

17. Sarrel, Sarrel and Nadelson, "Dyspareunia and Vaginismus," 9.

18. *Ibid.*, 10.

19. Prudence Tunnadine, "Balint and Vaginismus," *General Practitioner* (London), 21 November 1975, 16–17.

20. Sarrel, Sarrel and Nadelson, "Dyspareunia and Vaginismus," 10.

21. Bob Mandel, *Open Heart Therapy* (Berkeley: Celestial Arts, 1984), 61–2.

22. Musaph and Haspels, *Dyspareunia*, 28.

23. Masters and Johnson, *Human Sexual Inadequacy*, 245.

24. *Ibid.*, 245.

25. Leiblum and Pervin, *Principles and Practice of Sex Therapy*, 186.

26. *Ibid.*, 186.

27. Sarrel, Sarrel and Nadelson, "Dyspareunia and Vaginismus," 11.

28. Friedman, *Virgin Wives*, 134.
29. *Ibid.*, 129.
30. Elaine Showalter, *The Female Malady: Women, Madness and English Culture, 1830–1980* (New York: Pantheon Books, 1985), 75–8.
31. *Ibid.*, 75–8.
32. *Ibid.*, 129.
33. *Ibid.*, 132.
34. *Ibid.*, 195.
35. Orbach, *Hunger Strike*, 68.
36. *Ibid.*, 19 and 48.
37. *Ibid.*, 127.
38. Eichenbaum and Orbach, *Understanding Women*, 87.
39. Bezemer, "Vaginismus: A Women's Problem?," 1–2.

CHAPTER 4

1. *Woman's Own* magazine, "Discovering Your Body" (London: IPC Magazines Ltd., November 1986).
2. M. Scott Peck, *The Road Less Traveled* (New York: Simon & Schuster, 1978), 315.
3. Prudence Tunnadine, scientific director, Institute of Psycho-sexual Medicine, personal correspondence with author, London, 22 October 1987.

CHAPTER 5

1. Friedman, *Virgin Wives*, 138.
2. Masters & Johnson, *Human Sexual Inadequacy*, 244.
3. *Ibid.*, 244.
4. Thomas Kiernan, *Shrinks, Etc: A Consumer's Guide to Psychotherapies* (New York: Dial Press, 1974), 222.
5. Friedman, *Virgin Wives*, 62.
6. It is important to note that Freud's theory of psychological development and his observations about women's psychology and femininity have been commented on and reappraised by feminist psychoanalysts. As Eichenbaum and Orbach state in *Understanding Women*: "Freud's concepts were made through patriarchal spectacles, either unconscious of or unconcerned

about this bias. Thus, his theories relating to women's psychosexual development suffer from a particular narrow vision," 62.

7. Friedman, *Virgin Wives*, 84.

8. *Ibid.*, 84.

9. *Ibid.*, 101.

10. Joanna Ryan, "Feminism and Therapy" Pam Smith Memorial Lecture, May 7, 1983 (London: Polytechnic of North London, 1983).

11. Musaph and Haspels, *Dyspareunia*, 40.

12. *Ibid.*, 39–40.

13. *Ibid.*, 40.

14. Masters & Johnson, *Human Sexual Inadequacy*, 244.

15. Kaplan, *The New Sex Therapy*, 486.

16. Musaph and Haspels, *Dyspareunia*, 40.

17. Friedman, *Virgin Wives*, 105.

18. *Ibid.*, 33–4.

19. *Ibid.*, 33–4.

20. *Ibid.*, 105.

21. Patricia Gillan, Susan Golombok and Patricia Becker, "NHS Sex Therapy Groups for Women," *British Journal of Sexual Medicine* 7 (1980), 44–5.

22. M. Masud R. Khan, "Introduction," in *Through Paediatrics to Psychoanalysis: The Collected Papers of D.W. Winnicott* (New York: Basic Books, 1974), xi–xlviii.

23. Julia Segal, *Phantasy in Everyday Life: A Psychoanalytical Approach to Understanding Ourselves* (New York: Viking Penguin, 1985), 94–5.

24. *Ibid.*, 95.

25. D.W. Winnicott, *The Child, the Family and the Outside World* (New York: Viking Penguin, 1964), 27–28.

26. Kiernan, *Shrinks, Etc*, 214.

27. Leiblum and Pervin, *Principles and Practice of Sex Therapy*, 388.

28. Bezemer, "Vaginism: A Women's Problem?", 3.

29. *Ibid.*, 3.

30. Michael Gorkin, *The Uses of Countertransference: Working with the Therapist's Response* (New York: Jason Aronson Inc., 1987), 105–31.

31. Peter Rutter, *Sex in the Forbidden Zone: When Men in Power*

—*Therapists, Doctors, Clergy, Teachers and Others—Betray Women's Trust* (Los Angeles: Jeremy P. Tarcher, 1989), 159–91.

32. The basis for the ideas expressed in the letter can be found in Jeffrey M. Masson, *Against Therapy: Emotional Tyranny and the Myth of Psychological Healing* (New York: Atheneum, 1988). and *Final Analysis: The Making and Unmaking of a Psychoanalyst* (Reading, Massachusetts: Addison-Wesley Publishing Co., Inc. 1990).

33. Peck, *The Road Less Traveled*, 316.

CHAPTER 6

1. D.W. Winnicott, *The Maturational Processes and the Facilitating Environment: Studies in the Theory of Emotional Development* (Madison, Connecticut: International Universities Press, 1964), 51.

2. *She* magazine sex survey, "Who Does What and Where?" February 1987 (London: The National Magazine Company, Ltd.), 46–9.

3. John Bowlby, *The Making and Breaking of Affectional Bonds* (New York: Routledge Chapman & Hall, 1979).

4. Luise Eichenbaum and Susie Orbach, *What Do Women Want: Exploding the Myth of Dependency* (New York: Berkley Publishing Group, 1987), 194–6.

5. Jolan Chang, *The Tao of Love and Sex: The Ancient Way to Ecstasy* (New York: Dutton, 1977), 81–3.

6. Tunnadine, "Vaginismus," 17.

CHAPTER 7

1. Susie Orbach, *Fat Is a Feminist Issue: The Anti-Diet Guide to Permanent Weight Loss* (New York: Berkley Publishing Group, 1982), 130.

2. *Ibid.*, 131.

APPENDIX

1. Martin Weisberg, "Vaginismus," *The New Physician*, vol. 3, April 1982, The Student Medical Association, Schaumberg, Illinois, 29–31.

BIBLIOGRAPHY

Abraham, Hilda C. and Freud, Ernst L., eds. *A Psycho-analytic Dialogue: The Letters of Sigmund Freud and Karl Abraham 1907–1926*. London: Hogarth Press, 1965.

Balint, Michael. "Training GPs in Psychotherapy." *British Medical Journal*, vol. 1, January 16, 1954 (pp. 115–120).

Barnes, James. "Primary Vaginismus Part 1: Social and Clinical Features." *Irish Medical Journal*, vol. 79, no. 3, March 1986.

Berne, Eric. *A Layman's Guide to Psychiatry and Psychoanalysis*. New York: Simon & Schuster, 1968.

Bezemer, Willeke. "Vaginism: A Women's Problem?" Paper presented at Symposium Rutgers Foundation, Heidelberg, West Germany, June 1987.

Bowlby, John. *The Making and Breaking of Affectional Bonds*. New York: Routledge Chapman & Hall, 1979.

Chang, Jolan. *The Tao of Love and Sex: The Ancient Way to Ecstasy*. New York: Dutton, 1977. Available from Gower Publishing Co., Old Post Road, Brookfield, Vermont 05036, (802) 276–3162.

Draper, Katharine, ed. *Practice of Psychosexual Medicine*. London: John Libbey & Co., 1982. (May be ordered direct from John Libbey & Co. Ltd., 13 Smiths Yard, Summerley Street, London SW18 4HR.)

Drenth, Jelto J. "Vaginismus and the Desire for a Child." *Journal of Psychosomatic Obstetrics and Gynecology* 9 (1988): 125–137.

Eichenbaum, Luise and Orbach, Susie. *Outside In-Inside Out*. Published in the United States in an expanded version as *Understanding Women*. New York: Basic Books, 1984.

————. *What Do Women Want: Exploding the Myth of Dependency*. New York: Berkley Publishing Group, 1987.

Ellis, Havelock. *Studies in the Psychology of Sex*. vol. 3. New York: Random House, 1900.

Friedman, Leonard J. *Virgin Wives: A Study of Unconsummated Marriages*. London: Tavistock Publications, 1962. (Out of print.)

Gillan, Patricia, Golombok, Susan and Becker, Patricia. "NHS Sex Therapy Groups for Women." *British Journal of Sexual Medicine*. September 1980 (pp. 44–5).

Gorkin, Michael. *The Uses of Countertransference: Working with the Therapist's Response*. New York: Jason Aronson Inc., 1987.

Kaplan, Helen Singer. *The New Sex Therapy: Active Treatment of Sexual Dysfunctions*. New York: Brunner-Mazel, 1974.

Kiernan, Thomas. *Shrinks, Etc: A Consumer's Guide to Psychotherapies*. New York: Dial Press, 1974.

Knight, Lindsay. *Talking to a Stranger*. London: Fontana/Collins, 1986.

Leiblum, Sandra R. and Pervin, L. A. *Principles and Practice of Sex Therapy*. New York: Guilford Press, 1980.

Mandel, Bob. *Open Heart Therapy*. Berkeley: Celestial Arts, 1984.

Masson, Jeffrey M. *A Dark Science: Women, Sexuality and Psychiatry in the Nineteenth Century*. New York: Farrar, Straus & Giroux, 1988.

Masters, William H. and Johnson, Virginia E. *Human Sexual Inadequacy*. Boston: Little, Brown & Co., 1970.

Musaph, H. and Haspels A. A. *Dyspareunia: Aspects of Painful Coitus*. Translated by Marianne Loring. Utrecht: Bohn, Scheltema & Holkema, 1977. (Out of print.)

Orbach, Susie. *Fat Is a Feminist Issue: The Anti-Diet Guide to Permanent Weight Loss*. New York: Berkley Publishing Group, 1982.

————. *Hunger Strike: The Anorectic's Struggle as a Metaphor for Our Age*. New York: Avon Books, 1988.

Payer, Lynn. *Medicine and Culture: Notions of Health and Sickness*. New York: Henry Holt, 1988.

Peck, M. Scott. *The Road Less Traveled*. New York: Simon & Schuster, 1978.

Rutter, Peter. *Sex in the Forbidden Zone: When Men in Power— Therapists, Doctors, Clergy, Teachers and Others—Betray Women's Trust*. Los Angeles: Jeremy P. Tarcher, 1989.

Ryan, P. *Feminism and Therapy*. London: Polytechnic of North London, 1983. (Available from Department of Applied Social Studies, Polytechnic of North London, Ladbroke House, High-bury Grove, London N2 5AD, England.)

Sarrel, Phillip M., Sarrel, L. J. and Nadelson, C. "Dyspareunia and Vaginismus." In *Treatments of Psychiatric Disorders*. Vol. 3, edited by Harold I. Lief et al. Washington, D.C.: American Psychiatric Association, 1989.

Segal, Julia. *Phantasy in Everyday Life: A Psychoanalytical Approach to Understanding Ourselves*. New York: Viking Penguin, 1985.

Showalter, Elaine. *The Female Malady: Women, Madness and English Culture, 1830–1980*. New York: Pantheon, 1985.

Thompson, Clara M. *On Women*. New York: Basic Books, 1971.

Tunnadine, Prudence. "Balint and Vaginismus." *General Practitioner* (London) November 21, 1975 (pp. 16–19).

Winnicott, D. W., *The Maturational Processes and the Facilitating Environment: Studies in the Theory of Emotional Development*. Madison, Connecticut: International Universities Press, 1964.

———. *Through Paediatrics to Psychoanalysis: The Collected Papers of D. W. Winnicott*. New York: Basic Books, 1974.

———. *The Child, the Family and the Outside World*. New York: Viking Penguin, 1964.

Woodward, Joan. "The Diagnosis and Treatment of Psychosomatic Vulvovaginitis." *The Practitioner* (Birmingham, England), November 1981 (pp. 1–4).

Suggested Reading

The following are a selection of books which I found particularly valuable. Though not all relate specifically to vaginismus, there are areas in each that may have direct relevance to women having difficulties in relating intimately:

Women–Centered Psychoanalysis and Psychotherapy

Eichenbaum, Luise and Orbach, Susie. *Understanding Women*. (See Bibliography for details.) (New theories about women's psychology developed as the experience of two feminist psychotherapists. Illustrates case histories and centers on a radical reappraisal of the mother–daughter relationship and how it is affected by social conditioning.)

Mitchell, Juliet. *Psychoanalysis and Feminism*. New York: Random House, 1975. (A re-assessment of Freudian psychoanalytical theories in an attempt to understand the feminine psychology and oppression of women.)

Orbach, Susie. *Hunger Strike*. (See Bibliography for details.) (Very sympathetic and respectful approach to the anorectic's plight. Offers insights on how anorexia develops and guidelines as to the best therapeutic approach, including suggestions for self-help groups. Although this book is clearly not about vaginismus it is

the kind of sensitive and thoughtful study I hope one day will
be written by a therapist about vaginismus.)

SELF-HELP AND HEALING

Ernst, Sheila and Goodison, Lucy. *In Our Own Hands*. Los Angeles:
Jeremy P. Tarcher Inc., 1981. (Invaluable book showing how
self-help and therapy is within a woman's control. Offers comprehensive guidance on individual therapy, led-groups and self-
help groups with particular emphasis on feminist aspect.)

Hay, Louise L. *You Can Heal Your Life*. Santa Monica, CA: Hay
House, 1984. (Self-help manual, which firmly states that if we
are willing to do the mental work almost anything can be healed.
Offers practical steps for dissolving both fears and causes of emotional problems.)

Mandel, Bob. *Open Heart Therapy*. (See Bibliography for details.)
(Self-help book promoting attitudes and affirmations on how to
rediscover the inner love we all have. A list of professional Re-
Birthers is included at the back of book.)

THERAPY AND TREATMENT WITH THE CONSUMER IN MIND

Kovel, Joel. *A Complete Guide to Therapy: From Psychoanalysis to
Behavior Modification*. New York: Pantheon Books, 1976. (Self-
explanatory title and once called "The only credible consumer's
guide to therapy".)

Rutter, Peter. *Sex In the Forbidden Zone*. (See Bibliography for
details. Excellent ground-breaking book which explores the dynamics of power in male-female interactions and the tragic con-
sequences when those in power betray their trust. Offers
guidelines to protect women in intimate healing relationships, so
particularly relevant to vaginismus sufferers in treatment.)

UNDERSTANDING OUR EARLY DEVELOPMENT

Leboyer, Frederick. *Birth Without Violence*. New York: Knopf Inc., 1975 out of print. New translation from Ballantine Books New York due summer 1992. (Ground breaking book outlining the beliefs of an obstetrician that the emotional environment of birth has profound impact and life long effects.)

Miller, Alice. *Prisoners of Childhood*. New York: Basic Books, 1981.

———. *For Your Own Good: Hidden Cruelty in Child-Rearing and the Roots of Violence*. New York: Farrar, Straus & Giroux, 1983.

———. *Thou Shalt Not Be Aware: Society's Betrayal of the Child*. New York: Farrar, Straus & Giroux, 1984. (All three of Miller's books explore how society still sanctions child abuse so long as it is defined as "child rearing." Examines the unconscious need to repress early suffering, both by parents and therapists.)

GYNECOLOGICAL AND SEXUAL HEALTH

Brown, Paul and Faulder, Carolyn. *Learning to Love*. New York: Universe Books, 1978. (Sympathetic and down-to-earth self help guide with suggested exercises to help overcome sexual problems, including vaginismus)★

Delvin, David. *The Book of Love*. New York: St. Martin's Press, 1974. (Extensive information with sensitive drawings on all aspects of sexuality and sexual difficulties, including vaginismus)★

Dickson, Anne. *The Mirror Within*. London: Quartet Books, 1982. Available direct through Quartet Books, 27–9 Goodge Street, London W1P 1FD, England. Tel: 011–4471–636 3992 Fax: 011–4471 637 1866). (UK best-seller which looks, with humor, at basic assumptions and myths about female sexuality. Offers practical information to guide a woman through exploration of her inner feelings and her body.)

★These were the two books which helped me to diagnose my own vaginismus in the late 1970s.

Kitzinger, Sheila. *Woman's Experience of Sex*. New York: Putnam's Sons, 1983. (Includes sensitive photographs and drawings focusing on every aspect of sexuality from a girl through to womanhood. Vaginismus is included.)

Lauersen, Niels and Whitney, Steven. *A Woman's Body: The New Guide to Gynecology*. New York: Perigree Books, 1987. (Comprehensive reference book on all aspects of female health care, which aims to help women understand what goes on in the gynecologist's office for routine, and more serious, procedures.)

Nissim, Rina. *Natural Healing in Gynecology: A Manual for Women*. New York: Pandora Press in association with Methuen Inc., 1986. (A guide to help women care for their gynecological health in a truly preventative manner and offers alternatives from Eastern and Western cultures.)

Yaffé, Maurice and Fenwick, Elizabeth. *Sexual Happiness for Women*. New York: Henry Holt Publishers, 1988. (Very sensitive manual offering charts, questionnaires and programs to help discover a woman's sexuality. There is a self exploration guide with suggestions to overcome difficulties with penetration. Although written for women I think men would find this book immensely thought provoking!)

GENERAL HEALTH

The Boston Women's Health Book Collective (Details on pp. 273). is an excellent source for information on every aspect of women's emotional, sexual and gynecological health care, which houses materials from a range of sources not usually found in medical or public libraries. As well as publishing their now-famous *Our Bodies, Our Selves* (1971) they also produce, and regularly update, their own leaflets.

In March 1991 the author wrote an article titled "Vaginismus: A Personal Experience," which was accepted for inclusion in their new sexuality packet, a loose collection of articles to be available from the collective.

INDEX

McCartney, Marion, 135–36
males:
  domination by, 61, 91, 96
  effects of vaginismus on, 37–40, 83–84, 85, 87–89
  power of vagina and, 34
  sexual behavior of, 17, 33, 61, 83–86
  sexual problems of, 36, 39–40, 61, 83–86
  sexual stereotypes of, 85, 97–98
  see also fathers; sexual partners
Marnie, 18
marriage:
  annulment of, 50
  breakdown of, 39–40, 89, 137, 173
  conflicts in, 21, 36, 39–40, 89, 152
  dysfunctional, 19
  nonconsummation in, 33, 35, 37, 50, 88–89, 173
marriage counselling, 26, 106, 114, 274
massage, 128, 178
Masson, Jeffrey Moussaieff, 20, 91, 231
Masters, William H., 17, 23n, 25, 123–26, 137, 140, 183, 280
Masters & Johnson Institute, ix, 23, 25, 39–40, 83–84, 115, 123–26, 183, 185, 221, 227, 243, 271, 280
masturbation, 20, 27, 158, 184, 197
Mathieson, Anne, 30, 44–45, 73, 80, 86, 116, 142–48, 220
media, 96
medical histories, 175
Medicine and Culture: Notions of Health and Sickness (Payer), 207n
menopause, 13, 254
menstrual cramps, 207
menstrual periods:
  cultural attitudes and customs of, 6, 96
  shame and embarrassment associated with, 6–7
  see also tampons
Mesmer, Anton, 141
Metson, Kenneth, 174–78, 251–52
Mirror Within, The (Dickson), 34
mothers, 150
  child's internalized images and fantasies of, 64–65

daughters' relationship with, 6, 40–41, 48, 55–56, 61, 62–67, 71–72, 83, 92, 93, 98, 100, 159, 168–169, 170–71, 235, 237–40
fathers' relationship with, 7, 32, 66, 67, 161–62, 234–35
psychological needs of, 63
rivalry with, 66, 235
separation from, 62–63, 65–66
sexual attitudes conveyed by, 72–73, 92, 95–96, 100
surrogate, 56
Musaph, Herman, 179–81
muscles:
  relaxation of, 138
  spasm of, 9–10, 28, 160
  see also vaginal muscles

Nadelson, Carol, 19, 31, 57, 67, 281
narcoanalysis, 184–85
narcotics, 184–85
National Health Service (NHS), 271, 286, 289–302, 323–25, 327–29
National Sex Forum, 34
Natural Healing in Gynecology (Nissim), 176n
naturopathy, 177
New Sex Therapy, 136–37
Nissim, Rina, 176–77
No More Hysterectomies (Hufnagel), 99
nurse-midwives, 132–33, 249–50, 272–73
nurse-practitioners, 132, 133, 250, 272–73, 281
nurse-psychosexual counsellors, 132, 133, 134
nutrition, 178
nymphomania, 79

OB/GYN nurses, 132–36, 272–73
  doctors teamed with, 249–50
  training of, 133–34
Obstetrical Society (London), 16, 90–91
Oedipus complex, 66, 70, 157, 158, 163
Olsen, Kristin, 173
oral phase, 158